Jo Douglas read Psychology at Bristol University and after taking a postgraduate certificate in the teaching of infants and primary-school children, she gained her M.Sc. in Clinical Psychology at the University of Birmingham in 1975. She joined the Hospital for Sick Children, Great Ormond Street, in 1975 where she is now the Consultant Clinical Psychologist. She has had a wide clinical experience with children and families and is Director of the Day Centre for pre-school children and parents. Her present research interest is eating problems in young children. She has specialized in behavioural work with families and has written extensively for professionals as well as for parents. She has two children, Alexandra and Amanda.

Naomi Richman completed her medical training at St Hilda's College, Oxford, and at the Middlesex Hospital, London, and then went on to train in psychiatry at the Maudsley Hospital and in epidemiology at Columbia University, New York. She was medical director of a preschool day centre for children with developmental and behavioural difficulties and is particularly concerned about the problems faced by families with young children. She has carried out a number of surveys at the Institute of Child Health looking at the behaviour of young children, including sleeping patterns, ways of preventing sleep difficulties and of helping parents whose children are not sleeping well. Other research interests include the role of day nurseries and nursery schools in children's lives and the adjustment of girls in later adolescence. She now works for the Save the Children Fund in programmes to help children affected by war and conflict.

Penguin also publish a companion volume to this one, *Coping with Young Children*, written by Jo Douglas and Naomi Richman, and *Is My Child Hyperactive?*, written by Jo Douglas.

Jo Douglas and Naomi Richman

MY CHILD WON'T SLEEP

A handbook of sleep management for parents
of preschool children

Penguin Books

PENGUIN BOOKS

Published by the Penguin Group
Penguin Books Ltd, 27 Wrights Lane, London W8 5TZ, England
Penguin Books USA Inc., 375 Hudson Street, New York, New York 10014, USA
Penguin Books Australia Ltd, Ringwood, Victoria, Australia
Penguin Books Canada Ltd, 10 Alcorn Avenue, Toronto, Ontario, Canada M4V 3B2
Penguin Books (NZ) Ltd, 182–190 Wairau Road, Auckland 10, New Zealand

Penguin Books Ltd, Registered Offices: Harmondsworth, Middlesex, England

First published 1984
10

Printed in England by Clays Ltd, St Ives plc
Filmset in 9/11 Trump

*For our many friends who helped us
with their ideas and encourage nent*

Contents

Acknowledgements

We would like to thank our colleagues in the Department of Psychological Medicine of the Hospital for Sick Children, Great Ormond Street, London, for their participation in the development of this approach to managing sleep problems. We are especially indebted to Heather Hunt, who provided case material for the book, and to Ruth Levere and Richard Lansdown. The help of Heather Thorn, who typed the manuscript, is greatly appreciated. Finally, we are extremely grateful to the parents and children who attended the sleep clinic and gave their consent for us to describe the problems they have faced and overcome.

Chapter 1
Introduction

'My child won't sleep at night' is a heartfelt cry from many parents. The subject is an emotional one, and people tend to have strong ideas on how the problem should be approached. Swings of the pendulum in fashions of child-rearing leave parents feeling confused, not knowing whether they should be very strict and leave Jo or Kate to 'cry it out', or whether they should provide even more attention, take their children to their own bed or sit with them as long as they are awake. Some parents are filled with despair at the nightly dance of bed swopping and other complicated manoeuvres which develop in response to sleep problems.

Waking at night and problems over settling at bedtime are the most commonly occurring sleep difficulties in young children, and these are the focus of this book. At least one in five preschool children will present his parents with a major and persisting problem over sleep; probably a half to three quarters of young children at one time or another have periods of not sleeping well; and, as every parent has experienced, all babies have episodes of crying when nothing seems to soothe them.[1] This book is about what you as parents can do to deal with these upsetting problems.

The ideas in this book are based on our research into sleep problems, our experience of helping parents who came to a sleep clinic – or, as one parent expressed it, a 'sleepless clinic' – and the practice of one of us as a parent.[2]

We wanted to write the book because the problems are so common and so distressing, and because we felt that many people could be helped by the techniques we had developed if they had the chance to read about them.

Only you as parents can decide how you would like your child to sleep, but often it is difficult to know what you should do to achieve the desired night-time pattern. Once you have decided what you think is reasonable for your child and your family, the ideas we have been developing will, we hope, help you to achieve your aims.

It will become clear that we are in favour of routine and decisiveness as ways of promoting reasonable sleep patterns, and so we run the risk of being accused of insensitivity to the needs of children. In our work we found that the needs of *all* family members, parents and children, had to be taken into account when tackling a sleep problem. It may not be at all helpful for a young child to be in control of the whole family, with everyone running round him every night. But obviously you as parents will decide what is right and comfortable for you and your child. There is not just one 'right' way of responding.

We also feel it is important for both parents to participate in trying to solve a sleep difficulty. Fathers tend to get left out of discussions about young children, and yet they are just as important as mothers. If two people instead of one are involved in sorting out a problem, it can be much easier to deal with.

The book starts with an outline of what the condition of sleep actually is, and how children's sleep patterns develop. We then describe the different sorts of sleep problems that occur, nightmares, waking at night and so on.

The various explanations given for why children wake at night are discussed, including physical factors and family or social factors; and one chapter deals with crying and irritability in the first year and how babies can be comforted and encouraged to settle.

We then go on to suggest ways of coping with sleep problems. First of all we explain our general approach to managing sleep difficulties, and then we deal one by one with the various problems you may encounter. These include waking in the night, going into the parents' room or bed, and difficulties over going to bed or settling in the evening. There are also chapters on sleep problems in children who are still breastfeeding, and on helping children who are handicapped. The last chapter is about how you might promote good sleep habits in your child.

The first few years of life are a time of rapid change, and there is a wide variation in the amount of sleep children need and in their patterns of sleeping and waking. Waking is so common that it is perfectly 'normal' for a child to have unsettled sleep, and it does not mean that there is any underlying emotional problem. You as parents will decide what is a problem for *you*, and obviously families vary in what they accept and what they see as a problem that they want to change. If a period of unsettled sleep goes on for a long time this can have repercussions on all the family and there is no reason why you should not try to make things easier for yourselves, especially if you can be sure it will not harm your child.

The techniques we describe have been developed mainly for the one- to five-year-olds, but some of the ideas should be useful for older children; and we have a special chapter on settling babies (Chapter 4). Most people will probably not want to read the book straight through. If your child has a particular sleep problem you may want to look it up in the contents list and discover how we suggest tackling it. It is probably useful to read first Chapter 6, 'What can I do?', which is an outline of our general approach. In other chapters we have tried to cover most of the suggested causes of waking problems. If you have a young baby, try reading Chapter 4, 'Sleep in the first year of life', and Chapter 14, 'Can I help my child to sleep well?', which might give you some ideas on preventing sleep problems from developing in the first place.

If you belong to a parent group, it could be interesting to work through some of the chapters with the whole group. An alternative idea might be to develop a treatment plan with your health visitor, using our suggestions as a basis.

We illustrate the book with many examples of sleep problems we have been involved with and tried to help. The names and other details have been altered so that the individual families and their children cannot be identified. Although every child and every family are unique, there are often striking similarities in the sleep patterns of different children, and on reading these examples you may discover one which seems to be exactly like your problem. We hope this will encourage you to feel optimistic about the possibilities of change, and to have a go at trying our suggestions.

When talking about 'your child', we have given the sexes equal treatment by using 'he' and 'she' alternately.

Chapter 2
What is sleep?

Sleeping is a mysterious process. Why should we fall asleep every evening? And, once asleep, why should we wake up next morning instead of slumbering on for a few days? One result of sleep may be that it allows the various chemicals used by the brain to build up again ready for the next day's work; but this is only one aspect of sleep, and its nature is understood only to a limited extent.[1]

We do know that there are sleep centres in the brain which control its activity and the level of the mind's alertness. These centres determine the familiar adult rhythm of twenty-four-hour cycles of sleep and wakefulness – the 'circadian rhythm'. This twenty-four-hour biological rhythm is very powerful, although it can be overridden by other influences. If you have ever worked shifts you will know how hard it is to keep adapting to different time schedules and trying to remain awake at night; and sufferers from jet lag can take a week to adjust to a new time zone.

Light stimulation and the body's physical state can also affect a normal sleep pattern. In the Arctic winter, when it is dark all the time, explorers find that they sleep for longer periods, although their total sleeping time may not change. Young children can become quite confused by changes in the hours of daylight. In summer it can be hard for a two-year-old to get off to sleep whilst it is still light; when the clocks go back and the evenings are gloomy it may be easier for her to settle, although one two-year-old insisted on having a light in her room in winter because she had got used to falling asleep in daylight.

Sleep patterns can also be affected by various physical changes in the body; for instance, they may change as the levels of hormones circulating in the blood alter. The menstrual cycle produces changes in sleep patterns in some women as their hormones change throughout the cycle. A common pattern is to have a couple of days before a period when it is harder to sleep, followed by a few days of sleeping more than usual.

As we all know, psychological factors such as anxiety and excitement affect sleep. If you have an exam or are going away on holiday, you won't be surprised at not sleeping the night before. Anticipation of something exciting or worrying raises your level of alertness and makes it more likely that you will wake, though some fortunate people sleep *more* when they are anxious or depressed.

The sleep of young children is probably affected by similar influences to that of adults, although as yet we know less about this.

The nature of sleep

In sleep, the rational, thinking part of the mind is not active, and other processes of bodily functioning tend to slow down. The unconscious state is quite different: the unconscious brain hardly responds at all to outside stimuli, but during sleep the brain continues to be active in certain ways. Whilst asleep you are aware of the passage of time; you filter sounds from the outside world, and you respond to bodily states of discomfort, such as hunger, or to mental states, such as anxiety. As a parent you might sleep through a thunderstorm but wake immediately if your baby cries or stirs. In fact, both infants and their parents may well have a subtle awareness of each other's movements and noises; restlessness in either may disturb the other. However, during sleep and just after waking, the mind is much less alert than usual. Memory, decision-making and learning abilities are all affected. This obviously makes it more difficult for you to cope with night-time disturbances, to act rationally and decisively, and for your child to understand any complex reasoning about how she ought to go back to sleep or stay in her own room; so in the middle of the night it is probably not a good idea to get into long discussions with your two-year-old about why she has woken up.

Sleep has been divided into four stages, stage 1 being the lightest and stage 4, when it is most difficult to wake up, the deepest. During the night several cycles of sleep occur, moving from light to deep sleep and back again. (See Figure 1.) You are most likely to wake during light sleep (stage 1); probably most people, adults and children, wake or nearly wake on a few occasions every night. Unless we are anxious or excited or disturbed by some outside noise we drowse back to sleep again, and in the morning won't even remember that we woke. It seems that for many children with sleep difficulties, the problem is not so much that they wake up as that they do not slip back to sleep again, and require some external attention before this can happen.

Sleep has also been divided into 'rapid eye movement' (REM) sleep and quiet (non-REM) sleep. REM sleep occurs in

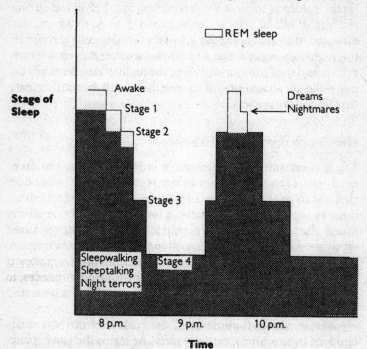

Figure 1. Stages of sleep.

the lightest stage, and this is the time when dreaming and nightmares are most likely. It is marked by an increase in body movement as well as by rapid eye movements.

It is possible to study sleep and waking in infants by making an electrical recording of brain activity. This recording or 'electroencephalogram' (EEG) shows the pattern of sleeping and waking, and the time spent in each stage of sleep. The recording will show what stage of sleep a child was in when she woke up. EEGs have helped to explain the differences between nightmares, night terrors and sleepwalking. There is still a lot that we do not know about sleep, and it is only recently that EEGs have been recorded in children who wake frequently at night for no apparent reason. Usually an EEG is combined with a record of eye movements, which increase during REM sleep and on waking. Another way of recording an infant's sleep is to have a video camera focused on her during the night whilst she is in her own cot. Activity meters attached to an arm or leg can give a record of overall activity in the night, showing when a child was awake. Babies are very active, and they move a lot during the night even when they do not wake up; so activity on its own does not necessarily mean that your baby is awake.[2]

How much sleep does a baby need?

There is considerable variation in how much sleep children need; but even newly born babies sleep less than was once thought to be the case. The idea of the passive baby spending most of the time quietly sleeping is far from reality. A study found that even immediately after birth the average time spent awake over a twenty-four-hour period was eight hours.[3] The amount of sleep gradually decreased until by sixteen weeks the average amount of sleep over the twenty-four-hour period was around fourteen hours and time awake was ten hours.

Just as in adults, the amount of sleep taken by the individual children in this study varied widely. At birth, the time spent asleep per day ranged from eight to sixteen hours.

Not only the time spent asleep but also the pattern of infants' sleep changes quite markedly during development. The amount of time spent in stages 3 and 4 of sleep is greater in infants and gradually decreases as they get older. This may explain their ability to sleep in quite noisy places. The older the person, the shorter the periods of deep sleep; old people spend very little time in deep sleep.

What are the effects of loss of sleep?

Many of you will have noticed that in spite of all the waking your toddler gets up in the morning full of life and energy. You are the one who feels exhausted and irritable. The fact that she is so happy is in itself a clue that she is probably not suffering from any lack of attention or security.

There is no evidence that wakeful nights have any long-lasting or serious physical effects on either children or adults. This is some comfort for those parents who have years of broken nights.

Studies of people whose sleep has been interrupted show that when they do fall asleep they make up lost time in two ways. They spend more time in deep sleep, stages 3 and 4, and also more time in REM sleep, as though they have to catch up on their dreams. Lack of sleep can have marked psychological effects. Some wakeful children are very irritable and whiny during the day. They look pale and tired, with dark rings under their eyes. These children may well be getting less sleep than they need.

Adults probably suffer more from lack of sleep than children. It is harder for them to cope, because unlike children they cannot have a few naps during the day when they feel like it, and they know that whatever happens they have to deal with all the responsibilities of daily life. Lack of sleep produces irritability and depression. You become slower at doing things, and it is harder to make decisions. Your actual judgement may not suffer, but reaction times are slower, and this can be important if you are driving a car or have to make snap decisions. It may be possible to carry on with routine activities, but anything that involves extra thought becomes difficult.

Chapter 3

Types of childhood sleep problems

The commonest sleep difficulties in young children are night waking and difficulties in settling at night, but it is quite likely that at one time or another your child will have other sorts of sleep problems such as nightmares and night terrors. This chapter describes the various types of sleep difficulty and the differences between them.[1]

Nightmares

Dreams and nightmares usually occur in the lightest stage of sleep, when the brain is still alert (stage 1). Research in adults shows that an external happening like hearing rain or some other sound influences the content of the dream or triggers it off, and this could also be true for young children, who once they start talking can often tell us about very simple dreams. It is not clear when children start having nightmares, but they may begin before the child can clearly talk about what he has experienced, and they almost certainly happen in the second year. They seem to be most common around three to four years, and there can be very few children who do not have them at some time. Immediately after a nightmare the child calls out and is obviously upset; he is fully awake and can remember the unpleasant experience, although young children may find it difficult to describe.

Nightmares are so frequent that on their own they cannot be considered a sign of emotional disturbance. Usually all that is required is comforting. You may find that excitement or watching television programmes seems to trigger them, and that a peaceful time before bed makes them less likely. Some children may be afraid to go to sleep because of the nightmares and may need extra reassurance then. A nightlight, a special toy (or even the cat!) can be a comfort.

If the nightmares are very frequent this may be a sign of generally high anxiety, and in that case you should look for signs of upset during the day as well. A bad run of nightmares will usually clear up spontaneously, but if not it may be reassuring to discuss the problem with your general practitioner (see the section on the anxious child in Chapter 5, p. 53).

> Four-year-old Jane was involved in a car accident. No one was badly hurt, but it was a shock for her. She developed a slight stammer and began having frequent nightmares. She did not like a nightlight because of the shadows it produced, but was comforted by a light on the landing and Snoopy the cat. It took two months for her to settle down. This length of time is not unusual, but her parents did begin to think she would never improve.

Nightmares are most common at the 'why' stage of childhood. Language is developing and children are beginning to question the world around them; it is a time of rapid learning, and your child may surprise you by the sorts of things he is turning over in his mind. If he is asking a lot of 'why' and 'what' questions during the day, about death, where babies come from and so on, an explanation which he can understand may help him to feel more settled at night.

Night terrors

In contrast to nightmares, night terrors usually occur in the deepest stages of sleep (3 and 4) and in the first few hours of sleep. They have been described as 'disorders of arousal'.[2] It seems that one part of the brain becomes aroused and more active, while the rest of the brain is still in the deepest sleeping state. Because the part of the brain related to awareness or memory is still 'asleep' the child does not remember anything about the episode next day, even though it can be very disturbing to his parents.

The part of the brain affecting expression of emotion is

active and the child looks as though he is having a terrible experience. The night terror is heralded by a blood-curdling shriek or a piercing cry, and when the parents rush in they find a child looking terrified, staring into space, perhaps sweating, possibly saying a few indistinct words. He is definitely not awake and will be very difficult to wake up, often just falling into a calm sleep if left alone. The best thing, in fact, is not to wake him but to wait for this calm state to take over, just tucking him up and making sure he is comfortable.

Night terrors look quite terrifying to parents, but they are rarely a sign of emotional disturbance, although they may increase at times of stress, for example, changing school. There is a tendency for them to run in families, and they occur more often in boys and in children between five and twelve years old. If they are very frequent they may be stopped by using a drug (diazepam) which decreases the amount of time spent in stages 3 and 4 of sleep. It is rarely necessary to use drug treatment, and most children grow out of night terrors. Fewer than 5 per cent of children seem to have them, and they are less common than nightmares.

Nightmares are usually easy to distinguish from night terrors because after a nightmare the child is normally awake or easily woken, and he remembers it at the time and the next day.

Sleepwalking and talking

These also usually occur when the child is in the deepest stages of sleep (3 and 4) and have some similarities with night terrors, in that part of the brain is 'asleep' whilst another part is active. The part of the brain controlling movement is active and that controlling memory and awareness is asleep, so your child is not in control of what he is doing. He may get out of bed and wander round the house, sometimes even into the street. But activities and speech are not really purposeful; he is not aware of what is going on and will not remember anything about it in the morning. He is difficult to wake and is best taken quietly back to bed. Children *can* hurt themselves by climbing out of a window or going into the street when they are sleepwalking, because they are completely unaware of their surroundings. It is very important to see that windows and doors are safely locked if your child sleepwalks regularly.

Like night terrors, sleepwalking is not usually a sign of emotional upset. Perhaps most children have an episode at one time or another, and it occurs regularly in about 15 per cent of children, more often in boys, and again it is something that tends to run in the family. It is more common in older children, from five to ten years.

Treatment is not usually needed, although certain drugs (e.g. diazepam) can be helpful, probably by cutting down the time spent in stages 3 and 4 of sleep. It may be a good idea not to make too much of sleepwalking episodes. The whole family can become very preoccupied with them, discussing them in great detail every morning. This can lead a child to feel very worried about himself or to start playing up because he knows his parents are worried about him.

> Nigel, aged six, had several episodes of sleepwalking, in one of which he gave himself a hard bang. His mother was going into his room several times a night to see if he was all right, and he began to ask if he could sleep with her. After an explanation to Nigel about the nature of sleepwalking, it was agreed that Nigel's door would be locked at night so that he couldn't hurt himself and that he was quite safe on his own. His parents reassured him that if he called out they would go to him at once.

Head-banging, rocking and other habits

Children develop a wide variety of habits to settle themselves to sleep – sucking their own or their mother's finger, stroking a blanket, twiddling hair – their own or someone else's. These habits seem to develop almost by chance because at one time they were found to be soothing. The soothing aspect may be related to touch (like soft, silky or furry textures), sucking something, or a rhythmic movement like twiddling a sheet or being rocked or patted.[3]

The disadvantage of sucking as a settling habit is that if it is a bottle or dummy or mother's finger, these 'disappear' during the night, and if the child wakes, someone has to go to him to give him the bottle or finger again. This is no problem if the child's own thumb is used, although it is thought that continuous thumb-sucking may push the top teeth forward.

A settling method which does not involve other people is the most convenient for the rest of the family.

Neil, aged four, could only go to sleep while twiddling his sister's hair. Gail was nine years old and certainly didn't want to spend thirty or forty minutes every evening lying down with Neil. It was not easy to get him to develop a new comforting habit so Gail could go off with her friends, but eventually he was quite happy with her woolly hat.

There seems to be an inbuilt mechanism for rocking or rhythmic movements to act as particularly good methods for soothing a baby.[4] We have largely given up using rocking cradles, but rocking in the pram or whilst being held are often used by parents. It is not unusual for children in the first year of life to rock themselves or bang their heads in their cot because they enjoy it, and these habits can become associated with settling to sleep. Some children rock so violently that they shake the bed, even moving it across the room, making a noise that the neighbours can hear; some bang their heads so hard they seem to be in danger of hurting themselves. Once well established as settling habits they can be very difficult to change, and it is certainly worth gently encouraging alternatives before rocking or head-banging becomes established. Changing from a cot to a bed may not stop rocking, but you will no longer have a cot flying round the room.

In some children, head-banging or rocking when settling to sleep or during the night is a sign of anxiety; signs of increased tension may be present during the day as well and may lead you to consider seeking further advice.

Rosalind, aged 2½, rocked her cot every night so loudly that the neighbours complained. This had started about two months previously and the parents realized that it coincided with a time when they were feeling particularly tense.

Rocking and head-banging occurring during the day with any frequency may be a sign that something is going wrong for your child. They may be temporary habits but usually they occur in young children who are miserable, bored or under-stimulated (see our companion book, *Coping with Young Children*).

Settling problems and sleep disruptions

By far the commonest types of sleep problem are what we have called 'sleep disruptions' and 'settling problems'.[5] These are the problems for which parents most often seek help, and for which we hope our ideas on management will be most helpful.

The term 'settling problems' refers to difficulties in getting a child into bed and settled to sleep in the evening. Some children stay up till all hours, eventually falling asleep on the sofa or going to bed with their parents. Others will settle to sleep only if a parent is in bed with them or after a long bedtime ritual which may last a couple of hours. Or once in bed the child may keep coming out of his room or calling his parents on all sorts of pretexts before finally dropping off to sleep.

Settling problems are common and, as you will know if this is a difficulty your child has, they can be very exhausting at the end of a hard day's work. You are unable to have any time to yourself in the evening and cannot arrange to go out because you feel a babysitter could not manage the situation. Some parents have to go to bed at nine o'clock or even earlier because their child will not settle without them.

Three-year-old Tom had never slept alone. He had a terrible temper every evening at about 8 p.m. about getting into his pyjamas. Sometimes his mother went to bed with him at 9 p.m. and they fell asleep together. Sometimes he stayed up all evening and fell asleep on the sofa. He always woke up when he was carried to bed and his mother then went to sleep in his bed.

The term 'sleep disruptions' refers to waking at night after having fallen asleep. As we mentioned previously, all children (and adults) probably wake fleetingly at some time during the night but most settle to sleep again. Only if the child cries for attention does a problem arise – not exactly one of waking, but of not being able to settle again without attention from parents.

Waking patterns are very variable. Mary called out to her parents several times a night, Steven only once; but Mary was always easy to settle with a drink and a cuddle, whereas Steven was awake for up to an hour. Eva went into her parents' room and wanted to stay; Angela wanted one parent to go back to her room and sit with her till she fell asleep again.

These patterns may often develop by chance, and a particular waking pattern does not seem to have any particular significance. In Chapters 4 and 5 we discuss some of the reasons which might cause a child to wake often or be unable to settle back to sleep again. About 20 per cent of one- and two-year-olds wake regularly, 14 per cent of three-year-olds and 8 per cent of four-year-olds.[5,6]

Occasionally it is difficult to know whether a child is waking regularly because of nightmares, especially if he is not yet speaking. It is unusual for a child to be woken night after night or several times a night by nightmares, and after a nightmare most children settle fairly quickly. If you are not sure if your child is having nightmares, it may be worth trying some of the settling methods described in Chapter 7 to see if they are helpful.

Martin, aged fourteen months, woke most nights yelling loudly and seeming quite upset. His parents tried cuddling and reassurance, but he usually took a long time to settle.

They worried that he might be having nightmares and were quite surprised that when they reduced the attention given to him when he woke, he began to sleep through.

Chapter 4
Sleep in the first year of life

The methods we describe for helping children to settle have been used mainly for one- to five-year-olds. It is less easy to know how to calm babies under one. The first few months of a baby's life are the most worrying for parents, especially with their first child. All sorts of experiences happen for the first time – the first sudden temperature, the first teeth coming through. Your baby can't talk and tell you what is the matter, and you may have sudden panics, feeling you don't understand what's going on.

This is often a time of great anxiety: your baby's behaviour can seem unpredictable, and you may be at a loss to know why she is crying and how to comfort her. This chapter describes some of the facts known about babies' sleep, which may help you when faced with a crying baby.

How sleep patterns develop

Recordings of babies' movements in the womb show that even before birth they have cycles of low and high activity; they are sometimes 'asleep' and sometimes 'awake'. After birth, cycles of sleep and wakefulness occur at short intervals throughout the day and night, with roughly the same amount of sleep (about eight hours) being taken in the daytime as at night. As the brain matures there is a gradual change in this pattern, and the baby begins to spend more time awake in the daytime and more time asleep at night. This change appears in the first few weeks of life. By sixteen weeks your baby will be sleeping twice as long during the night as during the day. By then, the average amount of sleep during the daytime is only four to five hours, but between 7 p.m. and 7 a.m. an average of eight to ten hours of sleep will be taken.[1]

The development of this daily or diurnal rhythm of sleeping

and waking depends on the maturity of the baby's brain, but it is also affected by what goes on around her.[2] For instance, clear differences between night and day, with a calm quiet atmosphere during the night-time and more excitement and activities during daytime, may help your child get used to this daily rhythm, and be more lively during the day and less aroused at night.

Out of each twenty-four hours, the new-born baby spends six to eight hours awake; so don't expect her to be asleep when she is not feeding; it is quite normal for her to be awake for an hour or so at a time. The span of time she can remain awake will gradually lengthen, from one to three hours at birth to about two to four hours at four months. The length of time she will remain asleep shows a more dramatic change. At birth she will sleep for at most three to five hours at a time and will then wake, probably because she is hungry. As the brain matures, she can remain asleep longer, and by four months she will be sleeping for six to ten hours at a time.

By three months about 70 per cent of babies are having their major sleep during the night.[3] This does not mean there is anything wrong with your child if she is not having six or eight hours' uninterrupted sleep by this age. As with the amount of sleep required, there are wide variations within the normal range, and some babies just take longer to develop a stable pattern of taking most sleep at night.

As the time spent asleep at night gets longer, the daytime naps get shorter, until by one year most babies are having two naps a day, one in the morning and one at some time in the afternoon or early evening. By this time the majority of infants are having a fairly long uninterrupted sleep during the night, although even at one year about 20 per cent will be waking regularly. Babies who begin to sleep through the night when they are between three and nine months do not always keep it up; so don't be surprised if your child, once a good sleeper, suddenly starts waking again. This was the pattern of sleep in one ordinary baby girl, Alex.

Alex was breastfed on demand. As soon as she came out of

hospital at seven days, she started having a long crying patch in the evening. Except when on the breast, she cried continually every evening from 7 to 10 p.m. This was a very stressful time for her parents.

At the eighth week she was becoming more settled. She was falling asleep at 8 p.m. and was then woken or woke about 11.00–11.30 p.m. for a breastfeed. She slept for approximately six hours and then woke again about 5.30 a.m. for another feed. By then she was taking about fifteen minutes to feed.

Alex slept in her parents' room for the first month and was then moved into her own room in a carry-cot. After the first few weeks she never fell asleep on the breast. She was changed before feeding, because she hiccupped a lot if it was done afterwards, and was put down to bed awake, taking only a few minutes to fall asleep.

At eleven weeks, it seemed that Alex was 'fighting sleep'. When she was ready for her midday or evening sleep she would become irritable and cry. Her mother used to pick her up but found that this just made the situation worse. She realized that Alex was getting over-excited and decided to leave her. This turned out to be a good idea, because after a little cry Alex would fall asleep.

From three months, Alex slept in a cot, and a musical blue-bird was played while she settled. She began to sleep through the night consistently at thirteen weeks. At first she was sleeping any time in the day between 11 a.m. and 4 p.m.; gradually the daytime naps concentrated to 10.00–11.30 a.m. and 3–4 p.m., and she was going to bed at 7 or 8 p.m.

Alex was breastfed on demand throughout. At five months she started on solids, and her last breastfeed was at nine months; she never had a bottle but started using a teacher-beaker at six months. Now she is two and a half years old and sleeps from about 6.30 p.m. to 7.30 a.m. She sucks her thumb as a comforter but has no special toys or blankets at bedtime.

Naturally, not every child develops a pattern as smoothly as Alex, so don't be too discouraged if things are not always easy. Every child is different; if your first child is difficult, maybe the second one will be easy. Don't lose your confidence in the first few weeks. Children go through phases and a baby who always seems to be irritable may suddenly enter a calmer, happier stage. Remember that the amount of sleep babies need is variable and that they often sleep less than you expect. Even new-born babies spend time quietly awake, taking in their surroundings and 'thinking'. At these times they do not necessarily need adult attention.

Why is my baby crying?

Many a parent driving round the streets trying to soothe their child or walking up and down the bedroom all night must wish we knew more about the causes of crying in the early weeks and how to help crying babies to settle. Nearly every parent has lived through the awful experience of not being able to comfort a screaming baby. She seems unhappy and uncomfortable, but nothing you do can soothe her. You are convinced she is not cold or wet or hungry, and can think of nothing else to try. Sometimes the onset of a cold or an ear infection explains the irritability; but often there is no apparent explanation.

Physical factors

The younger your child, the more likely it is that physical factors are causing the crying, although even in the first few weeks babies may cry because they feel bored and want some company. Crying is the main way a baby communicates her needs, and parents usually try to distinguish different cries for pain, hunger and distress.

Babies vary in their responses to discomfort and pain and in how much fuss they make when they are hungry (see the section on temperament, p. 40), and whereas one baby will cry loudly whenever she is teething or has a wet nappy, another will not be bothered. Below are some of the physical factors worth considering if you are not sure about the cause of crying.

Hunger

It can be difficult to know whether your baby is hungry, especially if she is breastfed and you can't tell how much she is getting at each feed. Mothers of first babies tend to feel unsure about feeds. One study found that second babies were fed more often and cried less.[4] You may find that more frequent feeds are helpful in soothing a baby who cries a lot, especially in the evening, when the reason may be hunger. This applies especially to breastfeeding (see the section on breast and bottle-feeding p. 37). By three to four months your baby should be able to go for about six hours at least without feeding during the night. Certainly by the first year a feed during the night should not be necessary; if your baby has an adequate feed before she settles down she is unlikely to get hungry till morning. The idea of night starvation is just a myth.

Discomfort

A wet or dirty nappy, or feeling cold or too hot, disturbs some babies much more than others. In general, they are more likely to settle if they are comfortable and warm.

Teething

From the middle of the first year, teething is a frequent explanation for waking. Like colic, it tends to be blamed for crying when there is no other apparent reason, but if your baby's gums are red and swollen you may well feel convinced that you have found the cause for her misery.

Illness

A child who is in pain, has a temperature, or is irritated by eczema will obviously wake more easily. A blocked nose due to adenoids or infection, or any difficulties in breathing such as asthma or bronchitis also interfere with sleep. Older children with various chronic illnesses or physical handicaps such as blindness are prone to sleep difficulties.[5] Deaf children take longer to get off to sleep; and children with autism or delayed development can be particularly difficult to settle at night-time.[6] Their sleep pattern can become completely reversed, with more sleep being taken in the day and long periods of wakefulness at night.

Even if your child has a physical problem which affects her sleep or makes it particularly hard to calm her, a change in your responses may do a lot to improve the situation and give you more energy for the daytime. (See Chapter 12.)

Colic

Colic is widely blamed as a cause of distress from birth to about three months, especially in the evenings. Dozens of explanations have been put forward as to the cause of colic, none of them substantiated; some people have even suggested that it doesn't exist! From their own experiences most parents probably believe otherwise. One problem in identifying colic is that babies often draw their legs up when they cry, so you can't be certain that this is a sign of stomach-ache. In one study, parents reported colic in 16 per cent of infants in the first year, mostly starting in the first two months; it was more common if solids were introduced in the first three months. It was not related to being breastfed or bottle-fed.[7]

Intolerance to cow's milk may be a cause of colic, and removing it from the diet might help.[8] But it is important to test this by carefully adding cow's milk to the diet as a 'challenge' to see if it does have any effect; otherwise you might embark on a difficult procedure quite unnecessarily. (See the section on allergies, p. 37).

It is known that cow's milk protein can be passed to a baby through the mother's milk, and in some cases withdrawing cow's milk from the mother's diet has apparently alleviated colic in breastfed babies.[9]

Breast and bottle-feeding

There is some evidence that very young breastfed babies are more likely to cry and be wakeful, especially in the evenings. It has been suggested that this is because human breast milk is less rich than cow's milk, particularly towards the end of the day. If the breastfed baby is fed on demand the problem will not arise; if she is fed on a strict schedule, then she might get hungry sooner than expected, especially in the evenings. In any case this will not apply after the baby is a few months old, because she is able to get more nourishment from each feed.

It can be difficult to judge whether your baby is hungry or is wanting to suck as a comfort. In Chapter 11 we discuss problems faced by mothers who have breastfed their babies up to and beyond the first year and find it difficult to wean them at night. Sleep is disturbed because the baby wakes several times a night wanting to suckle.

You can have the same problem, of course, if your baby wakes frequently wanting a bottle. In both cases the breast or bottle has become a habitual comforter rather than a necessary supply of food, and we discuss later how you can encourage settling and comforting habits which don't involve food.

Allergies and food sensitivities

Many parents are concerned that their child may be sensitive or allergic to various foods. Items commonly suggested are milk (human and/or cow's milk), eggs, oranges, chocolate, or any food containing colourings, flavourings or additives, especially tartrazine. Sometimes these foods are thought to enter the baby's bloodstream through breast milk. Overactivity, sleeplessness and generally difficult behaviour are believed to be produced by these allergies or sensitivities. In some children headaches, diarrhoea, vomiting and stomach-ache might also be explained by dietary factors. Children with eczema or asthma are sometimes allergic to certain foods, and in these children allergic reactions could also affect behaviour.

Our opinion is that at the moment it is very difficult to be sure how important this mechanism is as a cause of sleep disturbance. As far as we know, there have been no studies looking specifically at the effects of diet on sleep in young children; the experiments that have been done were concerned with older children described as hyperactive. The way such studies are done is to put the child on a very limited diet, containing none of the suspected foods, for a couple of weeks. The child is then 'challenged' by adding a suspected item of food to her diet. Her behaviour is observed before, during and after the 'challenge', preferably by someone who does not know what she is eating. This is obviously a laborious procedure.

Some studies have had positive, results, with an improvement in concentration and general behaviour when on the diet, and a reversal when challenging items of food are added.[10] Unfortunately, rather more studies have found no improvement from the diet.[11]

If you are convinced that your child is overactive and sleeps badly because of certain foods, then you may decide to try the effects of diet. Stomach upsets, diarrhoea and vomiting might be related to certain foods, and indicate which ones are to blame. Eczema or a family history of allergy may suggest that your child is allergic. We would suggest that you try our management advice first, because *most* overactive or sleepless children do not have any dietary problems and *do* respond to a change in management. A special diet is expensive and frustrating for your child, and requires an enormous commitment from you. In fact, some people have suggested that often it is this commitment which leads to improvement rather than the actual diet.

If you want to try the effects of certain foods you can remove each food from your child's diet for two weeks, keeping a record of her sleep. You can then re-introduce the food and see if there is a change in the sleep pattern; it may take some time before the effect shows. If you are considering cutting out cow's milk, for instance, you will want to be sure this is necessary before committing yourself to a long-term diet.

Some children who have been put on a special diet become undernourished because they are not getting enough or the right food. If you start a diet do make sure that your baby is getting enough to eat.

If you are breastfeeding you might consider whether you are having a lot of tea or coffee. It has been suggested that this can enter a baby's bloodstream through the milk and produce insomnia! One mother was having over twenty cups of coffee a day; when she cut down on this her baby certainly began to sleep better.

Birth and the early weeks

Wakeful children more often have a history of complications around the birth than similar groups of children who sleep well.[12,13] These complications include Caesarian section, raised blood pressure in the mother (toxaemia), a distressed baby during or just after the birth, heavy sedation during delivery. Of course, not every baby who has these experiences sleeps badly, and most poor sleepers have an uncomplicated birth.

Birth difficulties may predispose the baby to be restless and irritable, or in some cases they may be evidence that the baby was already unsettled before birth. Certainly a history of early irritability is more common in children who wake.[12–14] If your baby is very irritable or there were any problems around the time of birth, this may leave you feeling anxious and uncertain about how you are going to cope; and this will add to your difficulties.

The premature baby

Some premature babies sleep a lot, others are restless, and it is hard to predict how a particular baby is going to behave. Premature babies have to make up in their growth all the weeks they should have been in the womb. This means that they take longer to establish a diurnal or daily rhythm of being mostly awake in the daytime and mostly asleep at night. If they have to feed every three or four hours this will also shorten the length of time they can spend asleep.

Complications around the birth may increase irritability,

and on top of this, if your baby has to spend time in an incubator – which tends to be a rather bright, noisy place – she will not have had the chance to develop a calm routine by the time she comes home. You also will not have had time to get to know her, and it may take a while to feel confident in handling your premature baby, especially if she is very tiny.

The usefulness of developing a routine applies just as much to premature babies, but it is harder to know what to expect and when; so it is probably a good idea not to expect a settled sleeping pattern as soon as with other babies, and then you will be all the more pleased when it happens.

Temperament

There are wide variations in how much babies cry and how easy they are to calm. Part of the difference may be explained by the baby's temperament. Parents know that every baby is an individual, and the baby's temperament will influence the *style* of her behaviour, the way she does things. It could be that with some children you have to work much harder to establish sleeping habits because of their personality. For example, one infant will be much more active than another and, as we mentioned before, there are wide variations in the amount of sleep that children seem to need. Some babies are easy to soothe, and it is not difficult to know why they are upset. Other babies seem to get upset easily or do not respond readily when you try to calm them.

One study suggested that babies who wake regularly are more likely to be sensitive to stimuli and have lower thresholds of response to any stimulation.[15] These stimuli might come from outside the baby, such as noises or light, or from inside, such as being wet or hungry, or having wind.

Other studies find that some wakeful babies are slow to establish a pattern or rhythm in their daily activities. Bowel movements, hunger, appetite, as well as sleeping times, may all be irregular and unpredictable. Even though your child may be naturally slow in developing a diurnal rhythm or in set- tling, it is always worth trying early on to encourage a clear difference between night and day activities and to develop comforting settling habits right from the start.

A high level of activity has also been found to occur more often in children with sleep problems.[13] Certainly it is a help in older children if they have a chance to let off steam. It is often said that the active wakeful child is more intelligent than average. As far as we know, there is no evidence for this, although it is obviously a comforting thought in the middle of the night!

Emotional factors

It is a comfort if a physical cause for irritability can be found, but sometimes the cause may be emotional. Even very young babies, only a few days old, are sensitive to changes in routine or to situations of tension. The very first time you try to leave your baby for an hour or so, she may suddenly start to cry quite unexpectedly. If you are rushed or anxious or upset, your baby may well know. At other times over-excitement and getting worked up can cause irritability, and your baby may be able to calm down better if you leave her alone to settle.

It is difficult for parents to choose the right balance between giving attention when it is needed and overwhelming the baby with too much attention. There are wide variations in the amount and type of attention that babies like; part of the process of adaptation between parents and child that happens in the first months is learning what soothes your particular child.

Anna was a very restless two-month-old first-born. Her mother was at her wits' end because of her crying late into the night, and was walking around all evening with Anna in her arms. Anna was very active and responsive in the daytime. It was decided to see if giving her *less* attention at night would calm her. After a few nights' trial it was found that if well wrapped up in her cot and softly crooned to, she was able to settle fairly easily.

How parents affect settling

Parents often wonder how quickly they should go to their child when she cries. If they respond at once, will that encourage her to cry more, or will she feel secure and cry less? Evidence is conflicting. Some studies find that a prompt response produces more crying; other studies find the opposite. The problem is complicated because babies also influence their parents' behaviour.[4,16] The way they cry may make their parents more or less likely to come to them. What does seem important is the sensitivity or type of response that the parent gives. A quiet, confident manner is more likely to soothe the baby, whereas an uncertain one is more likely to rouse her. Parents who are 'over-responsive' and never give their baby a chance to settle alone may interfere with her learning how to settle.

> Tony's parents had waited a long time to have him, their first child, and he was born after a difficult forceps delivery. He was a poor feeder and his mother always went to him quickly at night in case he was hungry and needed to be fed. By the age of nine months he was a tubby little boy, used to four or five bottles of milk a night. His parents were exhausted by nine months of broken nights.

It is often difficult to know how to deal with a sleeping difficulty when it first arises. A cycle of wakefulness in your child and uncertainty of response on your part is all too easily established. Experienced parents usually find it easier to know the right moment to go to their child and the right amount of attention to give. Your first-born is more likely to have a sleep difficulty, possibly because you are learning this complicated process of responding sensitively.

Sometimes grandparents interfere with the natural development of parenting skills. A mother may feel undermined or 'on show' in front of her own mother and so may not react in the way she wants to; and inappropriate advice from well-meaning grandparents can be an obstacle to the growth of new parents' skills and confidence with their child. Of course, grandparents can also be immensely supportive and helpful, and many parents will gratefully recall the sensible and sensitive advice given to them in their early stages of parenthood.

Lots of people offer advice on how to help your baby sleep, from your next-door neighbour to your GP and health visitor. Unfortunately, these differing sources can be contradictory and may leave you feeling more uncertain than when you first asked for help. Moreover, external advice is based on other people's experience and rarely takes account of your desires or how you feel. For instance, you may desperately want to carry on breastfeeding your child, even though you are exhausted because you are woken so often at night by demands for feeds. Advice to parents must be tailored to their desires, so that they do not feel they are being forced to do something against their will. The odds are that no suggestions will succeed if parents do not feel confident.

Ways of soothing your baby

Many parents know instinctively that the best way to settle a baby is to use constant or rhythmic stimulation. They may pat, stroke or jiggle the baby, rock her in their arms or croon soft lullabies. Rhythmic sucking of breast, bottle, dummy or thumb acts in a similar fashion.

Results from experiments confirm what parents already know: constant or rhythmic stimulation, whether it be light, sound, warmth, touch or rocking, is the most effective way of quieting babies.[17] A record of the mother's heart-beat is usually very effective in young babies! A combination of several soothing methods is better than only one or two, as is shown by a well-tucked-up baby who is sung to and rocked.

Two methods of soothing, no longer in fashion, have been known for centuries – rocking cradles and swaddling.[18,19] Swaddling, where the baby is tightly bound in a woolly material, is possibly the most effective means of quieting. The baby is kept warm, has constant touch over most of the body, and has restricted movements of the limbs, so cannot wake herself up by moving too much. Another well-known method is carrying your baby in your arms or on your back. Babies in cultures where they are carried around on their mothers' backs tend to be quieter than the average Western baby. The skin contact with the mother's body and its warmth, plus the almost continual rocking of her body movements, probably all combine to quiet the baby.

If you can work out a quieting method which suits you and your child and stick to it, you will feel more confident about coping with times when she is upset.

Comforting habits

At around six months of age, babies begin to develop comforting or settling habits of their own, which in some ways replace those used by parents, and generally involve rhythmic stimulation.

Thumb-sucking starts even before six months.[20] It is not a sign of insufficient opportunity to suck; on the contrary, infants who suck their thumbs may have had *more* opportunities for suckling.[21] It is easy for the thumb to find its way into the mouth, and once the habit is established it is hard to break and may go on for years.

Other comforting habits shown by children include rocking, stroking something soft and twiddling someone's hair. Attachment to a special blanket or cuddly toy may begin at about six months.[22]

There is no evidence that the use of a comforting habit is a sign of anxiety, or even that it is a necessary stage of development.[23] On the other hand, once the habit is established it becomes a very important part of settling, as all parents learn if their child's special blanket disappears or disintegrates. It can be helpful to your child to have a comforter which can be used in times of upset, and although not essential it is a useful addition to a bedtime routine.

Can I help my baby to sleep well?

If you try to develop from the start a routine of settling your baby which she can get used to, this may stand you in good stead for the times when settling is really difficult. Most parents find that in the first few months they can take their baby with them when they go out in the evening and she will fall asleep easily. As long as you have some sort of routine at home there is no reason why this should interfere with sleeping, but as children get older it can become harder to settle them in a strange place.

A clear difference between day and night, between times for sleeping and waking, is important. When you are at home always put your baby to sleep in the same place, then try to see that she is not disturbed by what is going on around her. Keep the level of stimulation to a minimum, or you may interfere with settling. It is true that very young babies often seem quite oblivious to what is going on and will fall asleep anywhere, even at a party, once they are ready to sleep; but if you can practise developing a settling ritual whilst your baby is young it should be well established by the time you really need it. Babies fall asleep on the breast or bottle, and may eventually need to suck as a comfort before they can ever fall asleep. If you can, try putting your baby into bed whilst she is awake, so she gets used to falling asleep in her cot without sucking or being held.

We know the sorts of actions which are most soothing for babies (see the section above on ways of soothing). Try to find the method which suits your baby – singing, patting, rocking – but don't make it too complicated, or before long you will have developed a complex ritual which demands your presence for a long time. If you want to, you can encourage your baby to develop her own comforting habits such as a special blanket or toy. Give her a chance to settle. If she stirs or cries after your soothing, don't rush in, because you may wake her up just as she is dozing off. When they are falling asleep babies often make little jerky movements (as adults do when they are nodding off), and if you are not expecting this you may feel worried. Babies are active creatures; they move around a lot in their cots and often snore or snuffle. You have to get used to the noise and movement, otherwise you will be running in to your child all night.

It is probably a good idea to share the settling if you can, so that your baby does not come to depend on just one person; in any case, both fathers and mothers want to be involved in the enjoyable bedtime routine.

Try and find time to make settling a calm, pleasant experience for everyone. As you know, when you feel pressurized it is much harder to be comforting. The one night you decide to go out is bound to be the night she won't settle.

Chapter 5
Why is my child a bad sleeper? Family factors

The smaller families of nowadays often mean that until people become parents they never have to deal with a baby – and may hardly even have held one. It is not surprising that many parents feel unsure about how to manage bedtime and night waking. You may feel confused by conflicting advice from relatives, friends and 'experts' (like us!). Of course experts don't know your baby as well as you do, and as your confidence increases you will be able to work out how to manage things in your own way.

In practice we have found that generally it is not useful to delve back into the past or into the parents' or the child's psyche to find out the *cause* of a sleep problem. It is no good asking the child, because usually he doesn't know and the question makes him feel responsible for the problem. It is more profitable to concentrate on the here and now of how parents are responding at night-time and how that might affect the sleep pattern.

Parents' behaviour does have a strong influence on children, and this is the basis of our management approach. It can be difficult to recognize how your behaviour is influencing your child's behaviour, but we hope the chapters on treatment will help you to analyse your particular situation.

The family atmosphere

Children are very sensitive to their parents' moods and feelings and often respond by a change in their behaviour if there is any tension around. If you are feeling stressed your child may respond by not sleeping so well. If the stress is related to difficulties between you as parents, you may think your young child will not notice, but the chances are that he will. His waking at night and coming into your bed can be a way of preventing you from talking to each other and sorting out your problems, and his presence can act as a useful contraceptive. This may be what you want, but perhaps you have not realized how much you are involving your child in your affairs. We have found that having a child in their bed can also lead to a strained marriage if both parents are not in agreement about it.

Dawn, aged 3½, began to get into her parents' bed during the night, after they had quarrelled and were not speaking to each other. They thought that Dawn did not know about their quarrels, but were glad to have her there as this prevented further arguments.

Often parents who get on well generally just cannot agree about how to bring up their children. One parent wants to be strict, the other wants to be kind. They cannot agree on any consistent pattern and seesaw between two extremes. Obviously, this makes it difficult for a child to know what is wanted of him and in such a situation it is impossible to plan a night-time routine.

Four-year-old Tom's parents could not decide on a bedtime routine. He was put to bed at about 9 p.m., but always came downstairs again several times; his mother told him to go back to bed, but his father, who did not see much of him in the week, always wanted him to stay up longer. Eventually he got his way and stayed up. If his father was out, Tom refused to go to bed at all and often stayed up till midnight.

One parent may be able to deal with a sleep problem on their own but it can be impossible if their partner won't help or even seems to sabotage their efforts.

One-parent families

Single parents often have a tough time if they cannot share the responsibilities and worries of bringing up children. Night-time is particularly difficult; it can be lonely once the children have gone to bed, and a bedtime routine may never be established because they are allowed to stay up late for their company. It can also be hard to get out and difficult to organize babysitters, especially if the children 'play up' in the evening. So parent and children are very much thrown together, and a child can come to make ever-increasing demands on his mother's or father's time. If there is only one bedroom they may sleep together, perhaps in the same bed, because there is only one or because it is a comfort for both. This can make it even harder to limit the amount of interaction during the night.

With any child it is hard to draw the line between reasonable and unreasonable demands, between what you need and what your child needs. All parents must keep their own needs in mind; otherwise they can feel they are being swallowed up by their child's demands. Once you get resentful and then guilty about your resentment, it is not easy to have an objective, calm approach to night-time.

One single mother felt very guilty about leaving her children. They were aged two and four and kicked up such a terrible fuss whenever she tried to go out that she had given up asking a babysitter to come round. She was getting very depressed at never being able to leave the house, and as the children had no bedtime routine and went to bed when she did, she could not ask any friends round. The problem was solved by gradually establishing a bedtime routine and getting the children used to separating from her during the day (see our companion book, *Coping with Young Children*). She was then able to use a babysitter and have visitors in.

Sleeping alone or sharing a room

Gone are the days when most people slept two or more to a bed. Nowadays the majority of children in our society have their own room, or at least their own bed. Has this led to more sleep problems? It is hard to say, because sleeping alone is only one of the many differences in child-rearing between our society and other societies. In some countries children sleep with parents or another relative throughout childhood, and in these countries sleep problems do seem to be rare.[1] But these are usually extended families, with many adults sharing the care of the children, and presumably the parents do not demand the intimacy of sleeping just as a couple.

Paradoxically, because of these different social relations, sleeping together in traditional societies may make fewer emotional demands on parents and children than in our society. This may explain why in our society children who sleep with their parents, either from choice or necessity, are *more* likely to have waking problems.

Most couples now find they cannot sleep with a wriggling child in their bed and do want privacy, although some like the cosiness of sleeping together. There are all sorts of possible sleeping arrangements; it's up to you to choose the one you prefer. Children are adaptable, and there is no evidence that any particular pattern does harm, though once you have decided, it is important not to feel guilty or be indecisive about your choice. Some women who feel lonely when their husbands are on night shifts or away from home take a child into bed with them. This may be confusing if the child can't understand why sometimes he can sleep with Mum and other times he can't.

Being cramped for space can pose real problems over sleeping. Parents who have their child in the same room cannot control the night-time routine easily, and find it harder to limit the amount of attention or stimulation he receives. He may wake when they go to bed and then want to come into their bed; and it's hard to say no when you're all in the same room. If the child has already got used to sleeping in his parents' bed, it is harder to get him into a separate bed or cot.

We have found it possible for parents to put their child into a separate bed by gradually reducing the attention they give, and even to decrease the number of night wakings; but there is certainly no easy solution to this problem.

Brothers and sisters

Sleep problems are more common in only children, perhaps because the parents are not yet sure about how to settle them.[2]

Sleep problems also tend to run in families, affecting more than one child, so that the parents go without proper sleep for as much as four or five years. We have often helped parents to cope with a sleep difficulty in two children (see the section below on twins), and this can be very successful.

You may find your children sleep better if they share a room, although sometimes this just makes things worse because they run wild at bedtime or wake each other up during the night. There is no evidence that sharing has a good or bad effect on sleeping habits.

It's fun to share a bed or a room, and some children choose to sleep together. However, the decision is not always mutual; an older child may have to give in to a younger one, and this can present real problems at bedtime if one child does not want to go to bed alone.

Tim, aged four, always insisted that his sister, aged seven, went to bed at the same time as him. She wanted to stay up longer, and resented the fact that he always seemed to get his way and that she never had a special time for herself with her parents.

If one child is demanding at night-time, the needs of the others may be overlooked and it can be hard to strike a satisfactory balance.

The arrival of a new baby can have a marked effect on a child's sleep. He may refuse to go to bed, wake in the night, perhaps disturbed by your noise, or start coming into your room. It can be difficult to deal with this patiently when your nights are already broken by the baby.

Simone was nearly three when her brother was born. Up to then she had slept well, but she began to wake at night and go to her parents, wanting to stay the night in their bed. They used to take her back several times, and then her father stayed the night with her. Her parents had prepared her well for the birth and were upset at her response.

Simone's upset at the change in routine and the new arrival was discussed with her, and she responded quickly to a special time for herself before going to bed and a night-time management programme (see Chapter 10).

Twins

Twins seem especially prone to sleep problems. They often have difficult births and are unsettled in the first few weeks. It is harder to develop a routine with two babies, and as they are probably sharing a room, if one is unsettled or cries, this disturbs the other. As parents of twins discover, it needs considerable organization to develop a settling routine with two children. It can be convenient for each parent to settle one child, but this may end up with both parents involved in settling every evening, and this can be inconvenient. Similar problems can arise when you have children very close together in age. The techniques we describe have been used successfully with twins.

Pamela and Jane Green were aged sixteen months. They were born by Caesarian section and spent three weeks in an incubator. A regular settling routine had never been established and there was no regular bedtime. Between 7 and 9 p.m. they were bathed and then sat downstairs with their mother for up to several hours. They went to sleep between 10 and 12 p.m., and soon afterwards one of them, usually Jane, woke, and Mrs Green went to stroke her and give her a drink. Finally one or both of them came into the parents' bed. Mr Green did not agree with his wife's approach but had never been involved in putting the girls to bed.

The targets for treatment were to have a regular bedtime routine (Chapter 9) and to stop the twins going into their parents' bed (Chapter 10); and Mr and Mrs Green agreed that they needed to be more consistent. They carried out the treatment programme successfully over a period of two months.

Susan and Sarah, aged three, went quietly to bed after a bath, a story and a cuddle, and fell asleep quickly. They woke at

1–2 a.m. and Susan would run around the room playing while Sarah sat up in bed crying. This could happen two or three times a night, and it would be difficult to settle them again. They had always been poor sleepers and had been taking a sedative almost since birth. When they stopped taking it, they woke even more frequently.

The targets for treatment were to stop the sedative gradually, to limit the attention given on waking (Chapter 7), and use a star chart to encourage settling (Chapter 9, p. 90). It was difficult to get the two girls off sedatives, but this was eventually achieved after a month, and the parents were able to implement their plans to help the twins sleep through.

The effects of stress and the anxious child

Infants are very sensitive to their parents' mood. If you are depressed or anxious your behaviour changes in many subtle ways. You may think your children won't notice, but they probably will, and their sleeping could well be affected. So any upset in the family, or even at work, that affects you can affect them. You certainly can't protect them from these upsets, and with older children it may be a help to explain in simple terms why you are in a bad mood. Children often blame themselves for their parents' moods, or imagine something far worse than the actual truth.

Four-year-old Kim's grandfather had a heart attack, and an aunt was also ill. Her mother was spending a lot of time rushing around trying to deal with all the practical problems and give emotional support to her own mother. Kim's accustomed routine was broken and she began to have nightmares. Her mother gave Kim a simple explanation about the illnesses and took her to see her grandfather, who looked quite normal, and this helped Kim to feel calmer.

Children also have to face traumatic events themselves. Admission to hospital, separation from parents, illness, death, accidents, the birth of a new baby, may all disrupt a child's accustomed sleep pattern for a time. Although they may last for a few months, these disruptions are usually temporary, especially if you are able to be calm and reassuring. The difficulty is that they often occur when you yourself are already upset.

Liz, aged 2½, was admitted to hospital for an operation. When she came home she was clinging and demanding. She did not want to go to bed and woke in the night crying, although previously she had slept well. Her parents took her into their bed for a few nights and then got her accustomed to going back into her own bed.

If your child is having nightmares or wakes regularly, you will naturally wonder whether he is worrying about something. It can be difficult to know whether children are anxious, especially if they are not yet talking. Sometimes there seems to be no special cause for their worry; some sensitive children go through an anxious stage between three and five years. The worries seem to come out of the blue, and may be part of normal development, occurring as the child becomes more aware of the complexities of life. He may talk about some of these fears or worries during the day.

For no apparent reason, three-year-old Michael started having nightmares every night. He was a sensitive boy who did not like leaving his parents, and had fears of things like clocks, thunderstorms and loud noises. He asked questions about death and illness and needed a lot of reassurance.

It can be difficult to know how to reassure the anxious child and whether to take him into your bed. Most parents do take their child into bed at one time or another. Whether you do or not, probably the most reassuring thing for your child is for you to remain calm and confident. If you get too involved with the problem and keep asking him what he is worried about, this may have the wrong effect and increase his anxiety.

Other behaviour difficulties

Sometimes sleeping problems are only one of many difficulties; your child may be hard to cope with in the daytime as well as at night. Wakeful children can be irritable and whiny from lack of sleep. The situation then worsens if parents are also irritable from insufficient sleep, making it more difficult to have a satisfactory day and establish a peaceful night-time routine.

Parents sometimes expect too much rational behaviour and self-control from their young children; they think that as long as a child has plenty of love and attention he is bound to behave well. Perhaps your child needs more consistency and more guidelines about how you would like him to behave during the day as well as at night. A common reason for sleep problems is an escalating spiral of no limits during the day or at night, with exhausted parents and an increasingly confused child who would probably welcome more order in his life (see our companion book, *Coping with Young Children*).

A child with a difficult or sensitive temperament may find it hard to settle into a routine or adapt easily to changes.[3] This does not mean that no routine is required, and such children usually find it easier to cope when life is fairly ordered.

Children vary in their needs for stimulation and attention. You may be giving your child a stimulating and rich life, with lots of interesting experiences, but he may be getting over-stimulated. Most of us have probably experienced times when we have so many thoughts buzzing round in our heads that we cannot sleep at night or relax during the day. It is worth considering whether your child is in fact over-excited and might be calmer with somewhat less stimulation. A nap during the day and quiet times, especially before bedtime, help some children to calm down. Parents who don't see their child during the day tend to play exciting games in the evening. They leave it too late to have a proper winding-down time and then their child can't get to sleep.

The effects of stress on parents

Caring for young children is stressful in itself, and it is not surprising if at times it all seems too much to cope with. If you are also worrying about paying the rent or about your poor housing this adds to the strain. Women with young children are particularly likely to feel anxious or depressed; they usually have the main responsibility for looking after the children and running the home and they may also have an outside job. On the other hand if they are at home all the time they may feel isolated and lonely. Fathers too may be working long hours. Lack of sleep on top of all this can be the last straw, making parents feel that they can't cope or even that they may hit their child during the night.

It is not unusual to have these feelings, and most people who do manage to control themselves. But rather than trying to keep it to yourselves it is helpful to talk it over with someone sympathetic and see if there are any ways of making things easier. Obviously one way is to try and deal with the sleep problem, so that at least you can face the day feeling rested.

When to seek help

Talking over a problem helps to put it into perspective. Most of us can probably remember a worrying problem which disappeared after talking to a sympathetic person. Many parents are now in support groups which meet regularly. You may be astonished at how many of your group also have children with sleep problems. You can help each other by exchanging ideas on management or you may decide to tackle each child's sleep problem separately, using diaries and working out programmes as described in the treatment chapters. Perhaps you can find someone locally, such as a psychologist, social worker or health visitor, who will come along for one or two sessions to help your group get going.

Your general practitioner, health visitor or clinic doctor may also be helpful. Don't give up if they say you'll just have to put up with it; there may be somebody else around who has some ideas. There is an increasing number of people who are interested in helping parents with sleep problems and other behaviour difficulties in young children; for instance, some community psychologists and community nurses are experienced in this field.

If you feel at the end of your tether because of exhaustion, or because your child has a lot of other behaviour difficulties or seems very anxious, you may want to discuss this with someone experienced in child development. In the first place you could approach your health visitor, general practitioner, or the doctor at the child health clinic. As a last resort, psychologists or psychiatrists working in child guidance or hospital clinics offer help with the most difficult problems.

Chapter 6
What can I do?

Some children never establish a pattern of sleeping through the night; others start sleeping through and then begin to wake. In the latter case a particular event, for instance an illness or going away on holiday, may start the problem off, and then a pattern of disrupted sleep becomes established as a habit. Many explanations have been suggested as the cause of sleep problems. In our experience, the success of treatment is rarely influenced by whether you can identify a cause or not, or what the cause is. Probably in most children more than one factor has played a part in the development of a sleep difficulty. By the time you come to deal with it the original cause may well no longer matter, or you may never be able to decide what started it all off in the first place.

It is possible to help your child to settle or sleep through the night more peacefully, but it requires confidence and conviction that you want the situation to change. If you do not feel really sure that you want your child to go to bed at a set time or to sleep in her own bed, then do not worry about the problem; just accept it and enjoy the additional contact that you are having. But if it is really starting to irritate you, exhaust you or cause difficulties in your relationship with your child or your partner, then think hard about the possibility of change, using the ideas in this book.

The basic ideas of change

You may well have tried everything you can think of and found that nothing has any effect, or you may feel uncertain about how to carry out what you think you ought to do. We have discussed in previous chapters the many reasons why children are disturbed in their sleep. There comes a time when you suddenly wonder if you are contributing to the problem.

The basic idea behind our suggested approach is that reactions to a particular behaviour can often affect that behaviour. You know yourself that when something pleasant happens to you, you are likely to repeat the action that produced the good experience. The same happens with children. If their behaviour produces lots of attention and concern from you, this may actually encourage that behaviour to continue. This applies to daytime behaviour as well as night-time behaviour. We are not proposing a new or magical treatment, but just demonstrating how your common-sense approach to difficult behaviour during the day can apply equally well at night.

Night-time behaviour problems are not in any way different from daytime ones, although they often seem insuperable. You feel tired and less able to analyse and plan your own reactions, and many parents suffer very strong feelings of uncertainty and guilt about expecting their child to sleep on their own or sleep through the night without them present. Some parents are extremely worried that their child may feel rejected and cut off from them at night. This makes them run to every cry or whimper, and their strong parental feelings of love and care dominate their own needs for sleep and time to themselves in the evenings.

Many parents feel confused about the cause and effect of night-time disturbance, and the varieties of different reasons discussed in previous chapters add to the uncertainty about what to do. We hope to present a method by which you can attempt to sort out what is maintaining the pattern of disturbance. Once it is identified, you can then try to do something about it if you want to.

Here are a couple of examples that demonstrate how day and night-time behaviour problems operate in similar ways and how your reactions can interact with the child's behaviour to cause a spiralling effect of increasing difficulty. These are perhaps rather extreme examples, but not especially uncommon.

1. The child who whines for sweets

Your child knows from previous experience that sweets taste nice, and so when she sees them she asks for them. Sometimes you say no, because you feel it is bad for her teeth to have too many, but your child may persist in asking, because her desire is so strong. You may then again repeat no, and again she persists. By this time you may start asking yourself 'Is it worth an argument?' Or you may feel too busy to get involved in further discussion, or you may even feel annoyed that she is persisting. If at this point you say yes, you will avoid further upset and be rewarded by seeing your child happy. Your child will receive what she has asked for and be pleased with the result, but she will also have learned that she can get what she wants by persisting. So both parties are satisfied. If the pattern is repeated again in five minutes' time, you are likely to feel more resistant and your child will have learned to try harder. You can see how this interaction can spiral until you have your child whining and nagging and you feel angry and upset. Most parents will be able to stop this process before it becomes a problem, but we all know areas in our lives where we do not feel quite in control of our children's demands.

2. The child who will not fall asleep without you present

The same process can happen with sleep problems. Your child is highly rewarded by your company. Going to bed and sleeping through the night in their own bed is often the last thing children want to do. They know that you are going to leave them alone, and they will strive to keep your company as long as possible. Initially you may well have enjoyed this and found that encouraging your child to fall asleep in your lap was a pleasurable and rewarding experience. As the child grows older, you find that she does not fall asleep so readily and wants to play with you instead. You may then feel that putting her in her own bed to go to sleep is the way to limit her activity at this time of the day. This *may* work, but your child may cry desperately when you leave the room. You feel that your presence as she goes to sleep will encourage her to fall asleep peacefully, so you stay with her, holding her hand or stroking her, until she relaxes and falls asleep. This process can gradually lengthen, once the child knows you are going to stay. Many parents spend several hours in their child's room, often even falling asleep there themselves. As you know, it uses up your evening, you have no time for yourselves to talk or share experiences, and it can disrupt your marital life considerably. These other demands and needs can then make you begrudge the time spent getting your child to sleep and you begin to feel angry and resentful.

These two examples demonstrate how a problem can evolve from simple beginnings. Most parents never clearly think out their reactions to their children's demands, and the pattern evolves without any real plan. Often this is satisfactory and works well, but there are instances when it can go wrong and we have to take stock of what has happened and try to correct it.

The focus of change

The focus of change is clearly to look at ways in which you react to your child's demands at night. This is not to say you are to blame; rather the reverse – you are the one who can do something about it. Worrying will not make the problem go away and neither will searching for the reasons why your child doesn't sleep right through the night. The cause of the problem is not as important as what is happening now. You can change your response, and through that you can change your child's behaviour.

The techniques we shall describe in the following chapters will help you to change and think about what you are doing. We do not propose that this is how all children and parents should be, but have found this a method of helping certain parents change a state of affairs that has become distressing and upsetting to them and their child.

Sleep diaries

Keeping a sleep diary is an essential part of planning any change and should precede any decision to alter your reactions to your child's sleep habits. It is a simple method of keeping a clear record of what is happening at the present moment.

Our memories tend to exaggerate problems when we recall doing something we do not enjoy. In the morning we are notoriously unreliable at remembering what happened in the middle of the night! A sleep diary helps you record and remember precisely the sequence and duration of events. The aim is to have details of what is happening and your response to it every night. It must be written at the time the events occur, not the next morning; so keep it by your bedside with a pen at the ready.

Your sleep diary can be laid out as shown in Figure 2 (p. 63). It can of course be tailored to your needs; for example, if your child is difficult to get to bed but sleeps right through the night, you obviously will not need to record her night-time sleep pattern.

For a reasonably reliable sample of the night-time problem it is wise to keep this diary for one to two weeks before you consider changing your tactics. After two weeks you should have a reasonable picture of what is happening. Sometimes it is a surprise that the problem on paper is not half as bad as you had imagined. Sometimes the mere process of keeping a check on your child and yourself makes you alter your reactions slightly, so that your child gets the message and her night-time pattern begins to improve. Sometimes parents find that altering nap times has a big effect on settling in the evening.

If you are still worried and exhausted, now is the time to plan change, but it is vital to carry on with the diary to check whether your changes in management are in fact having any effect. The diary is a way of monitoring improvement and showing you how far you are succeeding with your plan of action.

	Monday	Tuesday, etc.
Time woke in the morning	6.30 a.m.	
Times and lengths of naps during the day	1.30 p.m. to 2.45 p.m.	
Time went to bed in the evening	8 p.m.	
Time settled in bed in the evening	10 p.m.	
Times and lengths of waking in the evening, and what you did	Stayed awake and cried when put to bed. I had to sit with him till he went to sleep, cuddling and playing.	
Times and lengths of waking at night and what you did	Woke 11 p.m.; settled 11.15 p.m. I went in and tucked him up. Woke 1 a.m.; settled 2 a.m. I went in, cuddled him, gave him a drink. Woke 4.15 a.m., settled 4.45 a.m. Husband went in, gave him a drink.	

Figure 2. An example of a sleep diary.

Setting yourself a target

The records in your sleep diary will give you clear information about what is happening. If you want to change this, then you need a goal to work towards. Writing the goals down can be a way of making you think hard about what you want to change, and in that process you will probably come to some joint agreement to have a go. We often ask parents to go away and discuss precisely what they would like to happen and plan how they are going to co-operate in this. Funnily enough, writing things down can often make you feel more committed to keeping up your change in tactics, so that you don't give up half-heartedly after two difficult nights.

Goals may vary from getting your child into bed and settled by 7 p.m., so that you can go out for a couple of evenings each week, to stopping the night-time bottles or having four nights out of seven undisturbed.

Discussion between parents can be a vital part of this process. A husband may decide that the problem doesn't really bother him, as his wife does most of the night-time care. If so, then they need to discuss whether he is going to be involved in the change pattern; if not, then he should not make comments to his wife that may undermine her attempts at change. He may suffer a few nights' disturbed sleep as his wife tries to get their child to settle alone instead of rushing in to cuddle her quietly back to sleep as she usually does. Other fathers are pleased to take an active part in the change process and may share or take over the settling procedures from their wives.

Thinking about the target of change is also a way of identifying a reward for yourself. If you specify that you would like two undisturbed nights a week, or that you want your bed to yourselves, then this shows what will be an incentive for you, so that you can keep up your efforts at helping your child change her sleep pattern.

Should I use drugs?

Even though many parents and doctors dislike giving sedatives and hypnotics to young children, they are very frequently used. Twenty-five per cent of children in one study had taken a sedative by the time they were eighteen months old.[1]

Considering how much these drugs are used we know surprisingly little about how effective they are. Do they really work? The answer seems to be that they may be helpful for some children, but for many others they are not. Children vary a great deal in their response to drugs, and it is often difficult to find the right dose. The same dose will have no effect in one child but in another of the same weight and age will produce sleeping all the next day. For some children, sedatives only make the situation worse: they may stay awake all night in an excited, 'drunken' state or they may be very irritable the following morning.

Even if a child's sleep improves when she takes a sedative, it rarely produces 100-per-cent unbroken nights. Wakings still occur, though perhaps less often or for shorter periods. We met many children in our sleep clinic who had been taking sedatives for long periods but still had a sleep problem.

Although there is no evidence that taking sedatives has any long-term ill-effects, as parents you will obviously not want to expose your young child to drugs if this can be avoided; and they should only be used for short periods.

If one sedative does not work, another may be helpful. You may find by trial and error that there is a sedative that helps your child to sleep better, and you may decide to keep this in reserve to use at times when you are completely exhausted or particularly need a good night's sleep.

We feel that in the long run it is more helpful to try out a management programme than to go on using drugs. Even when they help, they have only a temporary effect, and when you stop them the chances are that the sleep problem will return. If your changed management works, then it will be a permanent improvement. We have found that occasionally it can be helpful to combine a sedative with a management programme for a very serious problem, for instance, a child who is handicapped and is particularly difficult to calm (see Chapter 12).

The child with eczema often poses a worrying problem, because she gets so irritable and itchy at night. It would be worth discussing with your doctor how your settling techniques can be combined with any drugs that are used, and you may find that with a changed management programme you can even reduce the doses you are using.

Chapter 7
My child wakes at night

The child who wakes at night is a distressing and exhausting problem for parents. During the first year your baby is gradually settling to a night and day routine which will carry on into his toddler years. As we said in Chapter 4, children are so variable that it is not possible to say exactly when you can expect a routine to be established, and you should not be surprised if what seemed like a set routine becomes disrupted and you have to start all over again. Generally we do not give specific management advice to parents until the child is one year old because of the vagaries of the first year, although we have described in Chapter 4 how we think you can give your child the best chance to establish a sleep pattern.

A wide variety of measures is used by parents whose children wake at night, such as a drink, a nappy change or a cuddle. Other methods include walking and rocking, taking the child into the parents' bed and even taking him out for a drive in the car. Parents tend to try again measures that have succeeded in the past. In desperation they will go through a whole series of tactics in a set pattern each night in the hope that it will work. In fact, instead of the child's behaviour being determined by the parents, the parents' behaviour becomes controlled by the child's response to them, and it is sometimes astonishing to see the variety and idiosyncratic range of activities that parents have learned to send their children off to sleep again!

Amy's mother would beat a drum gently to send her one-year-old off to sleep at night, but if this did not work she would breastfeed her or take her into the parents' bed.

Elizabeth, aged seventeen months, would be picked up, taken into the living room and given up to five bottles of orange per night.

Quite often parents will have tried letting the child cry but eventually given up and gone in to see him. This may well have exacerbated the problem, as the child will have learned to cry louder and longer for the attention that he wants. A vicious circle can then arise, with the parents feeling angry that the child is screaming so much at night, and the child getting himself more and more worked up to achieve the result he wants. This is not a happy state of affairs and produces suffering for both you and your child.

Many parents come quite quickly to know the different cries of their children and respond accordingly. A distress cry is different from a demand cry, and if these differences are recognizable your job is much easier and feelings of uncertainty and guilt are less likely. But some parents may not be able to distinguish these cries, and all their child's crying distresses them markedly. Initial lack of confidence, and perhaps lack of mutual support between the parents, can often undermine the natural process of responding differently to the various cries. A pattern of over-reaction can arise in which you go to the child at every whimper, and then find that you never have a good night's sleep for years on end. Naturally you become exhausted and irritable, and your marriage as well as your relationship with your child can be seriously affected. Parents vary enormously in how they cope with loss of sleep. Some may become so desperate that they are afraid of hurting the child at night; others may decide not to have any more children. Once your child has a waking problem it is made worse because of your exhaustion, and you may end up feeling that every night is a chaotic battle, with calm flying out of the window. To make it worse your child may be angelically happy and energetic during the day, so that you feel you have no right to be angry with him.

The aim of change

Children go through different phases of sleep at night and are more liable to wake at some times than at others (see Chapter 2). As we have mentioned, it is probable that most children wake during the night but quickly drop off to sleep again because there is nothing to alert them to full wakefulness. When your child wakes and immediately cries, your hope is to encourage him to settle off to sleep again contentedly without your having to go to him. If he has learned that when he cries you will come and give him drinks or play with him, then he is likely to rouse himself to full wakefulness with the purpose of gaining that attention. Some people think that the answer to the problem is, therefore, to leave the child to cry himself to sleep. This is *not* our answer. The distress and anxiety that this type of advice imposes on some parents can be unbearable.

Methods of settling

There is a large number of ways in which you can settle wakeful children, and we hope to cover the most common of these in this section. We shall give examples of measures that have gone wrong and are adding to the problem, and shall describe the processes of correcting them.

Checking

Your natural response to a distressed or crying child is to pick him up and calm him by cuddling and physical contact. In some cases this extends to a couple of hours of walking around the house with him in your arms, repetitively pacing up and down the room, or taking him downstairs to play until he is tired enough to fall asleep again. All of these techniques are very demanding of your stamina and patience. Some parents take turns in staying up with the child so that each of them gets an alternate night's sleep. The toll this takes on health, temper and work is inestimable.

If your child demands nothing other than your contact when he wakes at night, you must set out to teach him to play quietly on his own in his cot. Your attention should not augment his night waking, and if left to his own devices he should be able to fall asleep again on his own. Clearly, you need to stop all the extended routines that have become established and start to develop methods that will encourage him to settle more quickly.

You know at what stage of waking you go to your child. Some parents go immediately they hear the first whimper in the hope of forestalling a full-blown upset; others will wait until they realize the child is fully awake and will not settle until they go in to see him. With the older toddlers, you may find them banging you on the head with a favourite toy at 2 a.m. ready to have a play.

The aim, therefore, is for your child to settle himself back to sleep on his own if he wakes during the night; and the procedure that we have called 'checking' encourages this pattern to develop.

The first step in the change process is for you to go into the child's room when he starts to cry, to reassure him, stroke him and tuck him down to sleep in a deliberate manner. A firmness of approach, without undue sympathy or contact, is necessary so that the child receives the message that he is not going to be picked up and should go back to sleep. You should then leave the room, even if he has not settled. If he continues to cry, you should wait for a period of up to five minutes, then return and repeat the same procedure. This should carry on until he settles himself down. Once children realize that they are not going to get out of their cots they normally fall asleep quickly.

If this pattern of 'checking' is repeated consistently each time your child cries at night, then he should learn within three or four nights that his crying no longer achieves the desired end of getting up.

The advantage of this system is that the regular visits reassure you that your child is safe and well, and he knows that you are nearby to answer calls. The major feature that is crucial to this approach is firmness of manner, so that he knows you mean what you say. Consistency of your reaction is also a vital component, so that he learns more rapidly. If one night he is picked up he rapidly reverts to his previous crying pattern, and much of the work that has been done to change the pattern will be rapidly undone. A golden rule to remember is: 'I must mean what I say.' Many mothers have commented that once they made up their minds about how to cope with the night waking, the problem resolved itself very easily. Sometimes the difficulty has been to stop husbands undermining their wives' attempts by telling them to go and comfort the crying child. Here we see the importance of both parents understanding and supporting each other in the process of change.

Many parents who have successfully carried out the 'checking' method have found that making up their minds that the child should not be picked up has been a crucial steppingstone. Once they were resolved, the implementation of the change was simple; and they feel as if the child had sensed that they had made up their minds and were going to be firm. Sometimes parents have suggested that the child must have heard the planning of the tactics during the session and are reacting to the psychologist; but we feel the important feature is that the child senses the feelings of confidence and assurance in the parents' attitude. We cannot emphasize this point enough, and it is the reason why any doubts on the part of the parents in implementing the change tactics need to be carefully examined. A half-hearted attempt can be more damaging to the state of affairs at night than leaving well alone. Parents who give up lose a lot of confidence in themselves and in the possibility of change; so you yourself must clearly want the night waking to stop and be prepared to do something about it.

Doubts can obviously be discussed, but the psychologist is in no position to persuade parents to follow advice they do not agree with. Some parents enjoy the contact and the demands on them by their children at night, even though they may be exhausted by them. They also may have at the back of their minds an age at which they can expect their child to settle; if so, attempts at change before this age are probably doomed to failure. Other parents voice feelings of guilt or lack of certainty about leaving children alone all night.

But a child who is happy and loved during the day does not suffer in any way when left to sleep peacefully on his own.

However, it is of course up to parents themselves to decide on this.

Drinks and bottles at night

A very common response to a wakeful child is to provide a drink or a bottle in the hope that this will satisfy a need and help him to settle to sleep. It is a leftover from the days of night feeds during the first four or five months, and if your child is continuing to demand this night drink after the first year and on into toddlerhood, then it has probably turned into a habit for both you and him. It is unusual for children to need more liquid unless the weather is very hot, and even then water is all that is required.

Sue, a fifteen-month-old only child of older parents, was waking on average twice during the evening and twice a night after her parents had gone to bed. She was being given a bottle containing a small amount of juice at least once a night. She was a frail-looking child with large blue circles under her eyes, but clearly very bright and advanced for her age. She was starting to talk and could ask for her bottle at night. The pattern of waking had carried on from babyhood and she had never slept through the night.

The parents had been advised by their GP to stop giving her a bottle, but they had been unable to do this and had sought additional help, as the mother was completely exhausted. The drink was successful, in that Sue settled quickly to sleep, so the parents were reluctant to stop it, as they did not know how else to help her settle.

We carefully discussed their feelings about stopping the bottle. Both parents agreed that it should be stopped and that they wanted Sue to sleep peacefully through the night. Our initial plan was to try to wean her off gently by reducing the amount she was given, but this was unsuccessful over a period of a couple of weeks; Sue would demand more to drink until she had her fill. As her mother was still unsure about her needing the drink, we suggested that she should be given milk instead of juice, to see whether she needed additional nutrition at night. This was not the case, as the change had little effect on the number of night-time wakings over two weeks.

We then agreed that the graded approach did not seem to be working, and the parents both suggested that they should stop the bottle completely and just settle her down with reassurance. Within a couple of nights, Sue slept through the night for the first time in her life, and after that the number of night-time wakings generally diminished until two months later she had developed a pattern of sleeping right through the night until the early morning, when she would wake at about 6.30 a.m., ask for a drink and then fall asleep again for a couple of hours.

This example demonstrates several features of change that should be examined:

1. Quantity of drink – often the amount given to a child can be gradually reduced, without his realizing, until the comfort of the beaker or bottle is all that is necessary. Occasionally this doesn't work, as in the above example.

2. Type of drink – fear of the 'night starvation' invented by advertisers can often lie behind parents' willingness to give drinks at night. The effect of a switch in the type of drink, from juice to milk or milk to juice, will clearly be demonstrated if there is a change in the number of wakings each night. Usually there is no basis to the fears, and parents are reassured by seeing that the number of wakings does not alter. A child who regularly drinks milk at night can be switched on to very dilute juice or water in a gradual process of 'weaning', and then the amount can be decreased as above.

3. Number of drinks – a child who is having more than one drink a night can also be helped to reduce the number of demands. Parents should agree how many he is to be allowed each night, and any additional demands will be managed by reassuring him and telling him to go back to sleep. The child should stay in his cot and the parent should settle him down quietly and then leave the room.

Who settles your child?

In some families the job of going to a crying child at night belongs to the mother; in others the load is shared equally between the parents. But there are some instances where a mother becomes so upset at her child's cries that she is unable to stop herself picking him up and comforting him. If these mothers come to us for help and clearly admit that they feel unable to carry out the 'checking' procedure described above, then we discuss whether the father should take over the responsibility for settling the child at night. Of course, sometimes it is the father who feels compelled to respond quickly to the child. This is always a sensitive situation and depends on mutual trust and confidence in the relationship. A co-operative partner can save the day and allow the other parent, be it mother or father, respite from the responsibility of night-time management of the child.

If it is the father who takes over, his reaction at night is an unknown quantity to the child, and so the established pattern is immediately weakened. For a child who regularly cries and clings to his mother and anticipates that she will cuddle and play with him, the father will probably be a different prospect. The father can then implement the checking procedure described previously and be firm and confident in talking to the child at night.

If this tactic is used, then clearly the mother must leave decisions to her husband and pass over total responsibility for night-time management. The worst situation is where she is getting anxious and upset and transmitting this to her husband, who thus is undermined in his autonomy and confidence. The wife must support his approach and encourage him to carry out the change procedure.

Charts and rewards

The older child who is able to talk can be approached in a different manner from the younger child, using his ability to reason and understand the consequences of his behaviour.

This method involves an agreement with the child to reward him for undisturbed nights. The child gains a reward for not calling out to his parents, and the parents gain a peaceful night. Some call this bribery and dislike it because it rewards a child for something he should be doing naturally. Bribery is in fact a process in which someone receives a reward for doing something illegal, wicked or immoral; and encouraging your child to sleep at night is none of these! The technique is a simple way of teaching the child the required behaviour, and involves providing an alternative reward to parental attention at night. In fact, the attention he used to receive during the night is shifted to the morning.

The process is relatively straightforward and should be tailored to the individual child and the speed of change that is expected. A child who is waking several times a night may not be able to achieve the aim of undisturbed nights immediately, and so would not earn any stars if the goal was for him not to call out at all. Some children, in contrast, can aim for this target straight away. The method is to choose the night-time behaviour that the child can manage and then give him a star to stick on his chart plus lots of praise and encouragement next morning if he has fulfilled the requirements.

Luke was a three-year-old boy who had continued to wake every night since birth, and his parents were disturbed at least once a night by him calling out. He was usually given a drink and then settled back to sleep relatively easily. He had been in a bed for eighteen months, and if his parents did not wake to his calls he would go into their room and wake them up. He was a very active and alert boy who asked lots of questions and loved to listen to stories.

Our aim was to encourage him not to disturb his parents at night. The suggestions to the parents included leaving a bottle for him to reach at night with a nightlight on so that he could find it, and he was given a farm chart with animal stickers as a reward. He could choose a sticker to put on the poster each morning if he had not disturbed his parents in the night.

The sleep diaries revealed that before any change was implemented he had woken his parents 75 times in 41 nights. When they returned three weeks later he had only woken them 21 times, and on ten of these occasions they had no contact with him. He would drink his bottle on his own and had been delighted with his poster. He had naturally become less dependent on the stickers after a couple of weeks and did not always demand to have them. The parents were very pleased with the change. Six weeks later the improvement had been maintained; he had had 26 sleep interruptions in 44 nights, but during this time had had a bad cold which disturbed his sleep. He had occasionally asked for a sticker, and the parents had developed a pattern in which they did not get up for him at all unless he came in and asked for a drink.

Follow-up five months later showed that there was no sleep disturbance at all.

An important aspect of this approach is that the child can see his success in concrete terms on the chart. Obviously it is vital that a star or a sticker should never be taken away once it has been given. It is not possible to take away good behaviour once it has occurred. If the child does not succeed in reaching his target for a few nights, then he should not be given stickers, but no fuss should be made about the setback. As soon as he starts to have peaceful nights he should be praised and congratulated warmly.

Nightlights and comforters

In some instances, part of the plan for managing night-time waking is to provide a nightlight for the child, so that if he wakes at night he can either locate a drink or find his toys in his cot to play with. The need for this can be assessed from the sleep diaries. Once the child is not calling out at night, the nightlight can be switched off to see if he really needs it.

Many children take a comforter to bed. Some choose a different toy every night; others have a special sleeping toy or doll to take to bed. Thumb-sucking is clearly a good settler, as the thumb is portable, easy to find and the child can't cry and suck at the same time! These are methods that children use themselves to gain comfort at night. Tom, a thirteen-month-old, settled at night after his mother bought him a lambswool fleece to lie on.

The suggestions made in this chapter are applicable to you only if you want to use them. They are not a prescription for how you *should* behave, but they may provide a guideline on how to get out of a difficult situation that is exhausting you, and they have worked well with parents requesting advice. If you do try to change your tactics, do keep accurate sleep diaries to record any change and do keep to one method at a time. Your child needs time to learn your new pattern of behaviour; if you change the way you behave every few nights, how can he know what to expect? Try the checking system for at least a couple of weeks before you abandon it.

Chapter 8
My child won't settle alone

Problems of settling to sleep alone are often the root cause of both night waking and settling difficulties. A toddler who is used to your presence while she falls asleep is unlikely to lie awake calmly in the dark if she wakes in the middle of the night. Her natural reaction will be to cry or call out for you to help her fall asleep again.

This pattern is often a carry-over from the early months of life when babies fall asleep at the breast or bottle and are then gently lowered into their cots without disturbing their sleep. Some parents never take the next step of teaching or expecting their child to fall asleep on her own and consequently never put her to bed awake. Others move one step to independence by sitting beside their child, stroking her, singing or reading stories until the toddler falls asleep.

> Graham, a 3½-year-old, was always put to bed by his father, who would spend up to two hours lying on his bed hoping that his son would fall asleep. This dramatically reduced his evening, as invariably he would fall asleep as well and his wife would have to come and wake him.

> Sally, a two-year-old, had never been left to go to sleep on her own in the evening, and her mother spent on average an hour each night reading stories to her until she fell asleep.

The one-year-old who won't settle alone

If you are having difficulty settling a one-year-old, then you have the advantage of a daytime nap to practise on! This is often easier than trying directly with bedtime or in the middle of the night, as you feel stronger and more alert by day.

If your toddler has a reasonably regular nap during the day and her pattern is one of falling asleep while being rocked or having a bottle or breastfeed after lunch, then you can start the process of teaching by putting her down in her cot while she is still awake but very drowsy. It is important that she should be conscious of being put down. Now you may be horrified at the prospect of upsetting a well-balanced pattern that you have established to keep everyone calm. Your toddler may well force herself to full wakefulness when you put her down, and then you despair of her ever having a nap at all. But think about the long-term gains rather than the short-term ones and see it as a period of relearning that can be tricky, but will avoid long bedtimes or wakeful nights.

If your toddler does wake fully as soon as you put her down, then two main approaches are possible:

1. Be firm in your manner, encourage her to go to sleep and leave the room. You can then implement the five-minute checking routine described in Chapter 7 (p. 68).

2. Stay in the room with your child, tell her to go to sleep firmly and kindly, and stand beside her with a reassuring hand on her. Don't at this stage pick her up or become involved in further contact if possible. Encourage her to calm down and then to lie down again, with you still in the room. She will eventually get the message and lie down, reassured by your presence.

Once you have managed this for the daytime nap, then you can progress on to bedtime and the waking periods during the night.

If you feel very bold you may be prepared to tackle all three occasions at one go. This is clearly going to be faster, but it can be a bit strenuous. If you are lucky your child will recognize your firmness of manner and settle relatively quickly, but in some instances it can be a struggle. You can understand that your child is likely to be upset if you change your normal pattern of behaviour, and she may well try to get you to revert to cuddling her to sleep. But if you are able to get over the first three or four days of resistance, then the problems will quickly dissipate and your toddler will learn to settle herself to sleep alone, secure in the knowledge that you are around. Your cuddles and rocking times are just as important, but they are not necessarily associated with falling asleep: they are pleasant and warm times together. Going to sleep can be just as peaceful and enjoyable when on your own after a relaxing cuddle and song.

Polly, a one-year-old, had never learned to settle herself to sleep. She woke as much as seven times a night and ended up in her parents' bed every night. She would fight going to sleep at bedtime and would kick and thrash for about ten minutes while being held in her parents' arms, fall asleep and then be put into her cot. Mother was encouraged to teach Polly to settle herself to sleep during her regular daytime nap, using a five-minute checking procedure. After three days of crying for about 30 or 45 minutes and then falling asleep, she suddenly accepted the new pattern and would fall asleep by herself with no difficulty.

Helping your child to settle without your presence in the room

If you are still at the stage of lying or sitting beside your child until she falls asleep, you may want to be able to leave the room so that she can drop off without your presence. If this is your problem, then there are two methods of change:

1. Tell your child, using your own terminology and pet phrases, that you are going to leave the room and that you want her to go to sleep. If she cries, implement the five-minute checking procedure (p. 68) until she falls asleep.

2. Use a more gradual approach to leaving. This will involve a staged process of moving further and further away from your child while she settles to sleep. An example could be:

(a) Sit beside the bed rather than on it.
(b) Stop touching or stroking.
(c) Move your chair a few feet from the bed; no conversation.
(d) Move your chair near the door.
(e) Sit outside the door.

Helpful tips are to try to avoid eye-contact and to pretend to be tired and close your eyes. This will avoid being sidetracked into 'interesting' topics of conversation. Your aim is to reassure with your presence, but to make clear that you want your child to go to sleep and playtime is over. Your calmness, firmness and persistence will soon get through, and your child will be able to settle peaceably to sleep, understanding what you mean.

Jenny, a twelve-month-old, had a regular night-time routine. This was supper, a play period, a bath, change for bed, a bottle in her bedroom and being rocked in her mother's arms for up to 45 minutes until she fell asleep. The whole procedure was exhausting her mother. In addition, Jenny was waking two or three times during the night, and her mother would try all methods to settle her, including breastfeeding and taking her into the parents' bed.

We planned to get a bedtime at 7–8 p.m. Her mother was to go through the normal bedtime routine but put Jenny into her cot to fall asleep and then stay in the room to write letters and read, but not to interact with Jenny. Within the following two weeks Jenny had learned to settle to sleep by herself and her mother was able to leave the room just before she dropped off.

Daytime weaning was completed at the mother's desire in preparation for night-time weaning from the comfort sucking. Also the mother was able to organize her evening better around bedtime by having a snack before putting Jenny to bed so that she didn't feel hungry and anxious about the evening meal.

The next stage of the programme was to treat the night wakings in the same manner as at bedtime. Mother was to settle Jenny back to sleep and then leave. If she was distressed her mother could stay, but not interact with her.

The mother's confidence increased dramatically over the next couple of weeks. She felt that she no longer had to rock Jenny to settle her; the bedtimes were vastly improved, and she had managed to stop breastfeeding at night. She had been aware that there had only been a minimum amount of milk and that the sucking was purely for comfort.

A couple of months later, the mother reported that she felt well able to manage any night wakings and that Jenny was able to settle herself to sleep.

Bedtime routines

This is the name we give to the sequence of activities that you go through to put your child to bed. Different families do this in a different order, but an example could be:

1. Bath or wash.
2. Change clothes ready for bed.
3. Late supper or drink.
4. Story or song in bedroom.
5. Tuck up in bed/cot and goodnight.

Usually this is a pattern that occurs every evening, so that your child learns the order of events leading up to bedtime. There are different variations of this that can lead to difficulty.

1. No bedtime routine

If your two-year-old is resistant to any preparation for bed you may be reluctant to try putting her to bed, as it will only lead to upset. Probably your child is falling asleep downstairs on the sofa fully dressed and you are having to carry her to her bedroom on tiptoe hoping she won't wake.

If this is the case then it is important to rethink how much control your child is having over you and whether you are content with this. It is possible to be able to get her changed and washed and then calmly prepare her for going to sleep in bed. If you want to change the existing pattern, then you need to plan the routine you want to establish, and decide at what time it is going to occur, giving yourselves an approximate time-limit in which the whole sequence will be completed.

You need to judge whether to give your child her supper before getting her into her nightclothes, or whether this is something for her to look forward to once she is changed.

Some parents don't want spilled food on pyjamas. Similarly, washing has to be planned, and if you are starting to clean your child's teeth then this has to be after the last milk drink or food. You need a gentle but firm approach to start a bedtime routine. Both parents may choose to be involved, or either one can take the responsibility. Many fathers enjoy involvement at this time of day, and it takes the load from the mother's shoulders.

Your child should feel as calm and relaxed as possible before you put her into bed, and a cuddle or a song can be soothing. But it is important to put her into bed awake so that she learns to fall asleep there rather than on your lap. You can stay in the room until she falls asleep as a first stage in the process of teaching her to settle.

2. Erratic bedtime routines

If you take your child everywhere with you in the evenings, keeping her up some nights and not others, then you are likely to pay the price of having a child who does not necessarily settle when you want her to on the evening you are at home looking forward to a session in front of the television. A change in pattern every now and again is not at all disruptive, as long as the original system is reinstated when normality returns. But the child who has never known a regular pattern is not likely to conform easily to expectations that suit her parents. This does not mean that she must go to sleep in her own bed at a set time after a set routine every night. Some children adapt well to a more mobile life where they sleep in a variety of different places as long as there is an element of consistency and pattern in who puts them to bed and how they do it. If a parent is reliably around at a regular time in the evening to go through the bedtime routine, then the child will feel secure even if she is in a strange environment.

This contrasts with the child who has been brought up with a consistent pattern and place of sleeping, then suddenly goes on holiday. The unexpected change can be disturbing for a few nights, mostly through curiosity and wanting to explore, rather than through fear. Parents can easily feel upset that their normally predictable child has started to show a disturbed sleeping pattern. Usually this will only be a temporary phase.

If you realize that you have an erratic bedtime routine with your child and you are having trouble getting her to settle to sleep on her own, then it may be important to plan a predictable pattern for a few months to stabilize the routine and allow your child to learn your expectations.

3. Extended bedtime routines

If you find you are reading your child four or five books, telling her several stories or having to sit holding her hand until she falls asleep, then you have an extended bedtime routine! The important feature of bedtime routines is that they should be finite, though without fail your child will try to make them infinite. 'Just one more story' or 'Just one more book' is a cry heard in many homes at bedtime. The problem comes in deciding which is the last one. Your relaxed and happy child can suddenly turn into a tearful and clinging baby begging you not to go. If you are quite content reading to her or staying until she falls asleep, that is fine; but if you find it is disrupting your life and you resent the time spent just sitting, it is possible to alter this pattern.

Knowing that you have given your child time for a chat about the day's events and had a pleasant time with a song and story before she gets into bed or while she is in bed, there is no reason to feel guilty about saying goodnight and leaving her to fall asleep alone. You need to be firm, and if you say it is the last story, it must be. If you start going back on your word you are teaching your child that 'This is the last one' means 'Well, perhaps just one more.' You create uncertainty in your child, who does not know where the limit is and how hard to push you to give in. If the limit is clear, then the last-minute pleadings and tears will not occur, since there will be no result from such behaviour.

Comforters and other toys to encourage settling

A rhythmical movement or sound is regularly associated with calming and settling crying babies in the first year of life. Quite often this pattern is continued by parents in the second and later years because they have never really tried or wanted to change it. As your child grows up, your expectations of her behaviour change, and so the techniques you used at an earlier stage often do not seem appropriate. Many mothers who don't mind breastfeeding or rocking babies under one year start to feel reluctant in the second and third years. Sometimes there is a need for an alternative, and thumb- or finger-sucking often takes over from suckling. A comforting toy or blanket may become an object of attachment, needed at night to help settling; some children adopt a special comforter spontaneously, while others never seem at all interested in them. Sometimes parents create the link with teddy or another toy by always putting it to bed with their child. Sometimes putting a cuddly toy in your child's arms will avert the problem of her wanting to hold your hand while she falls asleep.

Also useful are repetitive musical toys that can be hung on cot-sides or placed beside the bed. You start the tune as you say goodnight and then leave the room; with luck your child will have dropped off to sleep by the time the tune has finished. This kind of toy can bridge the gap of your leaving and be a comforting familiar sound associated with sleeping.

Chapter 9
My child refuses to go to bed

Bedtime is a difficult time of day, as you are usually at your lowest ebb, wanting to sit down and have a rest after the exhaustion of a hard day's work. Anticipation of a tussle getting your child changed and ready for bed can be daunting, and it is easy to feel irritable and short-tempered or just give up and let him do what he wants. Some mothers feel that their children should be in bed before their husband comes home, not only because of the time but sometimes because of the general extension of bedtime routines if the father comes in halfway through. Other mothers wait for their husbands to be home before they start putting the children to bed, as otherwise they would not see each other during the week. Some fathers like to put their children to bed as their major mode of contact on week days, and this leaves their wives free to see to a younger baby or prepare the supper. Parents with more than one child will find it helpful if both of them are available at bedtime.

Getting ready for bed with the preschool child need not be a struggle. If it is a dreaded part of the day, then allocate some more time rather than be pressured by the prospect of the potatoes boiling over for your own supper.

Bedtime can be difficult if you have other children waiting to go to bed; there never seems enough time to see to each of them individually. Playing around can sometimes be the last straw as you attempt to get your child changed and washed. Getting cross and irritable will rarely help this process, however, and you will end up feeling angry with a crying and resentful child.

Setting a bedtime

Bedtimes vary dramatically from family to family. Some parents set 6.30 or 7 p.m. as an aim for their toddlers, while others wait until the child is tired and then put him to bed. Consequently bedtime can vary between 5.30 and 9.30 p.m. The choice of pattern is up to you, and if you are content with the knowledge that you can settle your child with little fuss then you have no concern. If on the other hand you are desperate to get your toddler into bed at a 'reasonable' time and are finding it extremely difficult to settle him, then it is time to look at the methods you are using to get him to bed. The prospect of a lively toddler rushing around all evening wanting to play can be unbearable after a heavy day.

Graham, a sixteen-month-old, would go to bed between 9.45 and 10.30 p.m. His mother worked full-time, and during the day Graham attended a crèche, where he would sleep for two to four hours. His mother would collect him at 6 p.m., and he often dozed on the one-hour train journey home. She felt that he needed a meal in the evening, and she wanted a chance to play with him, so he would rarely be ready for bed before 8 p.m. His parents were very caring and concerned, but also felt guilty that they saw so little of him. Financial circumstances were very difficult, and so no change of work patterns was possible.

Graham appeared to be getting enough sleep but at the wrong times of day; so the first step was to reduce his daytime naps to a maximum of two hours and make a more regular pattern for him in the evening. Both parents were exhausted in the evenings and were aware that they were irritable and not responsive to him. They were keen to set an earlier bedtime at 7.30 p.m. and consequently organized themselves to allow this to happen. As Graham had a large lunch and tea at the crèche, his mother was encouraged not to give him another meal in the evening, but to provide a snack for him on the way home. This had the added advantage of keeping him awake during the train journey.

Once they had decided on this plan they implemented it easily. A five-minute checking plan was advised once Graham was in bed, but with the other changes to his sleep pattern during the day he readily fell asleep within ten minutes.

This case example shows the importance of examining your child's total sleeping pattern. Keeping a diary of all daytime naps can sometimes be very enlightening. You may see that it would be worth keeping your sleeping toddler awake during the late afternoon with a better hope of settling him earlier at bedtime.

Planning an earlier bedtime

There are two methods of planning an earlier bedtime:

1. A graded approach to bringing forward the bedtime over successive evenings.

2. Setting a time and then teaching your child to settle himself to sleep.

The choice of approach will depend on your own preference but will also relate to the reason why your child is staying up very late. If you have never set a bedtime, then you will never have attempted to get your child to sleep before he is totally exhausted, so it may be worth trying out this possibility straight away; you may be surprised to find that he actually settles with no trouble at all. If on the other hand you have tried to settle him earlier and have failed, then a graded approach would be more suitable. It gives time for your confidence in yourself to build up, and your child will not notice the gradual changes.

The process of setting a bedtime, whether late or early, and helping your child settle to sleep is covered in Chapter 7. You need to have a finite bedtime routine, and you must stay calm but firm. Once you have started on the new plan your consistency is crucial, so that your child can rapidly learn that you mean what you say. The graded approach involves establishing an initial bedtime quite late, close to the time when your child usually falls asleep. This sets the scene for you to indicate that it is time to go to bed and commence the bedtime routine at a point when he is ready to sleep. It is unwise to prepare your child for bed at 7 p.m. but then not put him to bed until 11. The changing and preparation should be linked to sleeping, so that your child can learn to anticipate the sequence of events.

Once you have managed to do this for a few nights with no real difficulty, then you can make bedtime half an hour or an hour earlier. Again once this is a reliable pattern the time can be moved forward until your chosen and ideal bedtime is achieved.

Mary, aged 3½ years, slept well at night but would not go to bed while her parents were still up. Sometimes she fell asleep on the sofa in the lounge, but usually she would go directly into her parents' bed when they retired for the night. The problem had started after a heart operation at 2½ years of age.

Her mother wanted her to be in bed by 8 p.m. and agreed to try a graded approach to changing the bedtime. Initially, a 10 p.m. bedtime was planned. Mary was to be taken up to bed awake, and firmly encouraged to fall asleep by herself in her own bed. A bedtime routine was established so that she was regularly changed and washed for bed; previously she had occasionally been put to bed in her daytime clothes.

Mary quickly accepted staying in her own room but would continue to call out for things she wanted, taking between one and 2½ hours to settle to sleep. Her mother was reluctant to make bedtime earlier at this stage, so she decided to wake her at 8 a.m. every morning, rather than leaving her to wake at 10 or 11 a.m., as had happened previously.

Four weeks later the pattern of bedtime and getting up was well established, and Mary was not leaving her room once she had been put to bed. The settling period had reduced to between fifteen minutes and one hour. She had also been given a musical lamp to encourage her to settle. At this point her mother agreed to set an earlier bedtime of 9 p.m.

Within four weeks this was also well established and

Mary was settling herself to sleep mostly within half an hour. A target bedtime of 8 p.m. was then set and achieved within another month.

The child who keeps coming down in the evening

Sometimes a child is relatively easy to get to bed but after a brief sleep, or as soon as he is left, will repeatedly come downstairs during the evening with requests for drinks and other excuses. You may try a couple of times to take him back and after no success may allow him into the lounge to watch television. Eventually when he is sufficiently sleepy you may be able to get him to bed so that he stays there.

There are two possible methods for dealing with this problem.

1. Taking the child back to bed

Your child will need to be taken back to bed firmly and calmly, with the minimum of interaction, every time he comes down. This can be a daunting prospect, as it may occur up to twenty times in an evening, but once you have started on this plan it is very unwise suddenly to give in. If you do, your child will have learned that perseverance pays, and you will have more difficulty the next time you decide to try again.

Try not to be sidetracked into a series of requests, and if possible do not let your child into the living room. If he wants to say something, then it should be done in his bedroom. If the problem is marked, then each parent should take responsibility for taking the child back on alternate evenings, so that there is no possibility of one parent being played off against the other. Some children will prolong the returning to bed by asking to see the other parent, and a seesaw effect can develop, with both parents losing confidence in their own personal ability to settle their child.

A calm and settled approach should be used in getting your child into bed and then any of the techniques mentioned in Chapter 7 (p. 68) can be followed.

2. Rewards

From about the age of three years it is possible to use a reward system, in which your child earns a token of some sort for appropriate behaviour. Star charts, transfers, and sticky pictures can all be used to help him learn to stay in bed in the evening.

> John and James, aged four and two years, were a handful in the evenings and at night. They kept coming out of their room all evening and did not settle until about 11 p.m. Their parents were uncertain how to handle their behaviour and felt that the boys were stronger than they were. Certain aims were agreed, which included setting an 8 p.m. bedtime, and for the boys to stay in their room and be quiet once it was bedtime. A bedtime ritual was established that involved getting changed, getting into bed and having one short story. They were then bid goodnight and told to stay quietly in their room.
>
> Bedtime was initially set at 10.30 p.m. and then gradually brought forward by twenty minutes every few days.
>
> John was given a star chart for staying quietly in his room, as it was thought that James would be quiet and go to sleep quickly if not disturbed by his brother.
>
> To everyone's surprise John responded immediately to the star chart and stopped coming out of his room. Both boys began to settle quietly and James went to sleep quickly. The use of the star chart was gradually stopped after three or four weeks. Both parents were able to be firm and gained confidence in their management methods during this process.

The reward technique allows you to circumvent the normal nightly battle and may save you from returning your child to bed all evening. You must explain the reason for the stars clearly, and if your child does come down, you must not mention them in a retributive manner. The idea is to give a concrete symbol that your child values. He should be excited by the prospect of earning the 'prize', but your praise and encouragement are a vital part of his enjoyment. The whole process is a positive one and should not be used in a threatening manner. If your child persists in coming down, then take him back regularly. If after a few days he has been unable to earn a star then reduce your demands. For example, if he comes down on average seven times an evening, set your first target as 'five times or less earns a star'. This allows your child to experience the reward and will help to motivate him to keep earning them. Once he has earned three stars successively, then reduce the target to once an evening. This process of gradual reduction enables your child to feel success, and you can feel pleasure in rewarding him.

Problems of going to bed are often linked to difficulties with settling to sleep, but on occasion they are the only substantial feature of difficult night-time behaviour. A habit develops that you put up with even though it irritates you, and you come to expect the battles or the nightly trips upstairs as a matter of course. It is in some cases a prolongation of the bedtime routine, and so your reaction will be important in combating it. The often-heard response of 'All right, come and have a warm cuddle' or 'Just wait until this programme is finished' is exactly what your child wants to hear and will encourage him to keep popping down.

Chapter 10
My child sleeps in our bed

Having your child in bed with you can be very cosy and satisfying but it doesn't suit everyone. You may have initially decided that you will all sleep together but now find it too disturbing to continue. Alternatively, the habit may have developed from the early breastfeeding at night, when you took your baby into your bed to feed and she ended up staying there with you (see Chapter 11). Although breastfeeding has now stopped she is still coming to bed with you. (If you are still breastfeeding and want to continue, then you need to think carefully about whether you are prepared to get up to do this at night.)

Another reason for trying to get your child into her own bed may be that you are pregnant and it is getting a bit of a squeeze having three and lump in bed all together, or you may realize that the expected baby is likely to be in bed with you because of feeding and so the older child needs to move out. This is not something to worry or feel guilty about. Children sleep happily on their own and you will not be depriving her of essential comfort and security. If her fidgeting in your bed at night is causing you sleeplessness, then you are going to be irritable and short-tempered the following day, which will affect your relationship much more seriously.

An important consideration about having your child in your bed is the effect on your sexual relationship. If one of you often has to change beds to get some sleep, then you need to consider the consequences for your marriage. Some families appear to play musical beds in the middle of the night; as the child comes in, one parent goes on to the sofa or into the child's bed.

There are many reasons why parents want a child in bed with them. For instance, some women want their child with them for comfort while the father works late or is on a night shift. In other cases the presence of a child can be a useful contraceptive by preventing sexual relations. Before you decide to change your sleeping arrangements it is worth considering carefully what you would really like.

There are two main arrangements that can cause parents concern:

1. The child comes in during the night to sleep in their bed.
2. The child refuses to go to bed in her own bed but is put in the parents' bed and stays there all night.

The methods of changing these types of behaviour are slightly different.

The child who comes into your bed during the night

Your child may settle to sleep in her own bed in the early part of the evening and be perfectly content to stay in her own bed in her own room at this point. But when she wakes during the night her immediate reaction is to get out of bed and go into your room. Some more agile children can climb out of a cot, and parents are often understandably worried that they might slip or fall.

One technique often mentioned to stop your child changing rooms is to shut either her bedroom door or your own. This can work if the child is able to get back into bed, but where she has to climb back into a cot it is not so suitable. Some parents fear that the child may feel shut in if her door is closed, and yet if they close their own there is the danger of her wandering around the house at night. In some instances, children have collected a pillow and blanket and made a bed for themselves outside their parents' bedroom door.

> Tony, a four-year-old, would regularly leave a sleeping bag in his parents' room and sleep beside their bed, as they would not let him into the bed.

The other problem about closing doors is that the child may cry and become very distressed at not being able to reach her parents. This will create more disturbance and upset during the night than letting her into your bed.

The reasons and patterns for coming in at night are as varied as the manner in which different children do it. Some immediately wake their parents for a cuddle, while others slip in unobtrusively on the side of the heaviest sleeper. Parents who are not disturbed initially but wake up at some point and just find the child in bed with them often have the greatest difficulty in getting her back to her own bed. A simple method to help you wake as your child enters your room is to attach some bells to the doorhandle so that they ring when it opens.

Another consideration that should be mentioned is that some bedwetters will go into their parents' bed once they have wet their own, and unfortunately may then wet that bed too.

There are two possible techniques for changing this pattern.

1. Taking the child back to her bed

The main method for encouraging your child to sleep in her own bed is regularly and firmly taking her back to her bed as soon as she comes in. This should be done with the minimum of fuss and contact. She should be reassured, tucked up and then left to go to sleep on her own. If she returns, then she should be taken back again immediately. This can recur many times during the night and is an exhausting process for you. Because of the demanding nature of this pattern, both parents should agree on, and stick to, the contract of returning the child to her own room. If either of you gives in, it easily weakens the resolve of the other and makes the task that much harder. If your child just once achieves her aim of getting into your bed, then all your previous attempts to stop this will be nullified, and any successive attempts to change the pattern will be all the more difficult. One simple rule often suggested to parents is 'Let her in first time or not at all.' This is the reverse of the situation where the child has learned to persevere at getting into her parents' bed because she has experienced that sufficient attempts will succeed. It is clear that if she has to try six or seven times before she gets in, then she will do that to achieve her aim. If you are really too tired to take her back to her bed repeatedly, then she should be allowed into bed on first request, and later, once you have regained your strength, you can try again.

Firmness of resolve is essential, as it is the foundation of most child management. Once the child realizes that you mean what you say, the task of management is one-hundred-per-cent easier. Often we have found that, once parents agree on taking the child back regularly, the problem they thought insuperable is resolved within a few nights.

It is often helpful if it is the parent not usually involved with the child at night who takes her back to her bed; but sometimes parents alternate in this rather exhausting task. Holidays or weekends can be a good time for starting this change of routine, so that as you take your child back to bed for the ninth time you do not feel stressed by the anxiety of work next day. In the morning you can bring her into your bed for a cuddle; it must be clear that it is you and not your child who decides on this, but cuddling in your bed is a special privilege which need not be denied even if you are trying to get your child to sleep in her own bed.

2. Charts and rewards

Another approach with the three- or four-year-old is to provide a reward or a star on a chart if she stays in her own bed all night; or, if that is too difficult at first, she can earn a star for going back to her room quietly or for coming in only three times instead of six. This procedure was discussed in the previous chapter, and similar principles apply here. A contract is agreed with the child that whenever she sleeps all night in her own bed she will receive a sticker or a star to stick on the chart on her wall in the morning. These can accumulate to give a gold star for, say, three nights of sleeping alone; or the child can save up stars for a special outing or a surprise present.

This process helps defuse some of the antagonism and frustration that you feel at night, and your child is presented with a positive way in which to change.

John was a 3½-year-old who had shown marked problems at night. He would get up on average twice a night and go into his parents' room. He would settle quickly if allowed into their bed, but would take up to an hour to settle if taken back to his own bed. The parents had adopted a pattern of taking him in with them until he was asleep and then transferring him back to his own bed. On the second waking they would let him stay with them. Mother occasionally went to sleep in John's bed.

The problem had started when John was just under two years old. His father went into hospital for three days, and John slept in his mother's room whilst they stayed at her parents' during this period. The sleep disturbance continued, as his mother had another baby a few months later and he was left with his father for two months while she was in hospital.

They had tried medication to help John sleep, but this had no effect. They were both feeling quite desperate.

Advice centred on taking John back to his own bed every time he came into his parents' room; if he continued to be upset, a regular checking procedure was to be implemented by his father. John's night-time disturbance was resolved within a month of his parents starting to change their response.

Carl, a 2½-year-old, was regularly put to bed in his parents' bed and then transferred to his own bed in their room after he had gone to sleep. If he woke at night he would get into his parents' bed and stay there for the rest of the night, but he was restless and disturbed his parents' sleep. They were keen for help and wanted Carl to be able to settle to sleep in his own bed in his own room for the whole night.

The first plan in treatment was to change Carl's habit of creeping into his parents' bed at night. This was done by providing a little surprise of a wrapped sweet or cheap toy under his pillow in the morning if he had stayed in his own bed all night.

If he did try to get in with his parents, he was to be taken back to his own bed before he could get into theirs. Within four weeks the new pattern had become well established.

He was settling in his own bed and had only gone to his parents' a few times.

The final plan was to get him into his own room. Therapy finished before this was possible, as his room was being decorated, but he was looking forward to sleeping there and had already chosen a special nightlight.

The child who will not sleep in her own bed at all

This pattern is often linked with difficulties in getting children to bed at all. Sometimes it may develop when a baby wakes during the night and is taken to her parents' bed for comfort, and then they start to put her to bed directly in their bed because it saves them getting up later. In other cases it may have developed because the parents tend to let their child fall asleep in the living room or on their laps and then take her to bed with them when they retire for the night.

Rose, a 3½-year-old, would stay awake in the evenings and go to bed with her parents late in the evening. Her sleep problems were part of a difficulty in getting her to bed, but the result was that she stayed most nights in her parents' bed.

Some parents allow their child to stay in their bed all night because they cannot face the prospect of trying to get her to go to her own bed. Others try to take the child back to her own bed once she has fallen asleep, but invariably she wakes up just as she is being put down.

There are two main methods for resolving the difficulty. One is to move your child's cot or bed into your room and encourage her to go to bed in it while you sit close by until she goes to sleep. Preparation for, and talk about, her going to her own cot is important. Sometimes buying new bedclothes or putting a special toy in her bed which can only be played with there can help your child become interested in the idea. Some parents have tried initially to encourage the child to take daytime naps in her own bed and build up to sleeping there at night-time too. The child's bed can later be moved into her own room and the process of settling and comforting repeated in the new surroundings.

> James was a 32-month-old son of very young parents. He had recurrent chest infections and had been a difficult sleeper from the beginning. He would fall asleep on the sofa at about 8.30 p.m. and was then taken up to the parents' bed, where he would stay all night. This was seriously affecting their marital life.
>
> The initial plan was to encourage James to go to bed in his parents' bed rather than falling asleep downstairs, and both parents were to take turns at putting him to bed. This was successful, so the next stage was to put him in his own bed in the parents' room. Finally his bed was moved into his own room, where he had some surprise new bed-linen. The whole process took about three months and was entirely successful at the end of the treatment and at a four-month follow-up review. The parents now felt confident about handling James despite their youth and other difficulties.

If your child seems able to tolerate the idea of going to her own bed in her own room, then there is no reason why you should not try her there directly, rather than following the more gradual approach we have mentioned above. The idea is to encourage her firmly to stay there, and, once the decision is taken, not to put her to bed in your bed at night ever again.

You can build in as many rewards to this approach as you like, as long as they are linked to your child settling to sleep in her own bed. Your attention is very important, and you can have a special bedtime cuddle and play only if she goes to her own room. If she wants you to stay beside her until she falls asleep, this is fine initially and can gradually be eliminated later on. The final step will be to encourage her to fall asleep without your presence in her room (see Chapter 8). Her own room should be made as attractive and as comfortable as possible. It can be helpful to play fun games of pretending to go to sleep during the day.

As we said at the start, you need to think clearly about why your child is in your bed. If you are happy about it, that's fine. If you are concerned about it and are losing a lot of sleep or having to swap beds, then it is worth considering whether you really want your child there. There is nothing wrong with wanting the privacy of your own bed, and your child will not be damaged by sleeping in her own bed in her own room.

Chapter 11
Breastfeeding the night waker

Some parents continue to breastfeed into the second and third year of life and are perfectly content with this arrangement. The mother may enjoy the prolongation of the breastfeeding and feel pleased that the suckling at night is a comfort to her toddler.

Other mothers feel that breastfeeding up to one year of age is enough, and they begin to want some independence from their child after having provided so much attention and care for the whole of his first year. This first push towards personal independence and autonomy is an important phase for both mother and child. It is a natural phenomenon that is perfectly age-appropriate at one year as your child becomes more independent. He still needs you as a secure base and comforter for all of his problems, but breastfeeding does not necessarily have to be part of this. Your loving, cuddling and playing are sufficient for his emotional needs and sense of security. He will not be damaged if you decide to wean.

The issues surrounding breastfeeding can be complicated when combined with a night-waking child or one who sleeps in his parents' bed. It is difficult but possible to carry on breastfeeding an older child at night but reduce the number of night wakings.

David, aged twenty months, was breastfed seven times a night and always slept in his parents' bed. The parents had liberal attitudes and lived in a collective house. They did not want to wean David or change the sleeping arrangements, but wanted the mother to be able to have more undisturbed sleep. She was losing, on average, four hours' sleep per night.

The aim was to reduce the frequency of night feeding by teaching David to fall asleep without the nipple. He had always fallen asleep while on the breast during the day and the night. The parents eventually managed to teach him to fall asleep after a breastfeed rather than just leaving him attached to the breast.

There was a consequent reduction of feeds to about three per night, which entailed a loss of half an hour or one hour's sleep. At a follow-up interview four months later there had been a few spontaneous feeding-free nights, and the parents were then prepared to consider letting David sleep in his own bed.

This case example shows that, no matter what the parents' child-rearing philosophy is, a change of management can help to resolve difficulties. In this instance it was possible to reduce the number of breastfeeds at night without weaning or with-holding the breast. It is important to make a clear distinction between suckling and falling asleep, so that the two are not irrevocably entwined for your child. If you can do this, then he will stop using your nipple as a dummy that aids sleep. Feeds can be just as comforting and pleasant for both of you if you put him down to sleep while he is still awake after the feed. If you have never dared to do this before, you may dread the possible consequences. But you may find, to your surprise, that your child accepts the slight change in pattern perfectly easily. If he does complain and becomes upset, then perhaps you need to think about your settling procedure (see Chapter 8).

Weaning

Many parents with a night-waking child want to wean and yet feel unable to. Mothers may resent always having to be the one to get up, and they will be looking forward to the day when the load can be more equally shared.

Weaning can be the first major step in changing the night-waking pattern of your child, and as always it is easier to start during the day.

Edward, at eighteen months, had never slept through the night. On a bad night he would wake every couple of hours and be breastfed. He was also breastfed during the day at all mealtimes. His bedtime was at 8 p.m., and he would usually settle to sleep on his own after a brief cry. His father was able to settle him at times, usually in the early morning, when he would go into bed with Edward so that the mother could have some sleep.

The mother was very keen to wean, but attempts had failed. We planned a weaning schedule of breastfeeding Edward during the day after meals rather than before, and aiming to drop the lunchtime feed by this method of eating first. At night-time, the parents decided that the mother should breastfeed a maximum of twice and then let the father settle Edward at other times by pacifying him and then by a procedure of checking.

Within a couple of weeks this new routine was well established, and waking had dropped to once or twice a night. The parents were reluctant to push their luck, so the situation was allowed to stabilize over the next two weeks. Breastfeeds were at breakfast, bedtime and twice at night. The next plan was to drop the 4 a.m. feed and the bedtime one. The mother preferred this because she thought Edward was most keen on his morning and midnight feeds.

Two weeks later, despite some illness, Edward had managed five undisturbed nights, and on other occasions he was waking only once at night and once in the evening. All of the night feeds were then finally dropped so that he only had his one morning feed. The improvement in his sleeping pattern continued.

In this case the father's role was very important in supporting his wife's desire to wean and being prepared to help settle his son so that his wife did not have to face a battle for the breast in the middle of the night. It is possible for a mother to manage on her own if she wears a well-done-up dressing-gown so that her child cannot help himself. The difficulty is the emotional tie and the 'let-down' reflex as you comfort your child and try to get him to sleep. If your feeding pattern is well established and balanced, you are likely to have tender and full breasts for the first few nights as you reduce the number of feeds, so you are having to manage your own body and its physical reactions as well as the emotional demands of your child.

Facing the final feed

Some mothers who manage to wean their children during the daytime with little difficulty lose their confidence at night. They know that their child is merely comfort-sucking and is receiving only the minutest quantity of milk at night. If you are one of these mothers then it is important for you to consider carefully your feelings about weaning. You may say that you want to stop but still feel sad deep down at the end of this phase of babyhood. That is nothing to hide or feel ashamed about, and if you admit it to yourself, then you can put away thoughts about what you *ought* to do and do what you *want* to do.

If on the other hand you are starting to resent the situation and feel that it is out of your control, then you can easily lose confidence in handling your child. His demands for the breast become too emotionally laden for you to manage, and you can see no other way of getting him to sleep. It is important to have an alternative plan of action in your head, as once you have decided to stop night feeds it would defeat the whole exercise if you offer the breast again in desperation. You need to consider your settling regime, and plan how to teach your child to fall asleep off the nipple. You know that if he gets upset or hurts himself during the day you *can* calm him down without suckling. This applies to night-time too; breastfeeding is not the only answer to night waking.

Chapter 12
My handicapped child won't sleep

Mental, physical or medical handicaps in your child can interfere with your confidence in your normal parenting abilities. You may well feel a need to over-compensate for your child's particular handicap. This is also often tinged with guilt, and you may find yourself unable to set the limits and expectations that you would for other children.

The difficulties in sleeping patterns that we have discussed in earlier chapters all apply to handicapped children: they wake at night; they can be difficult to get to bed and settle to sleep; they may come into your bed. The problems are the same as in normal children, but often your anxiety about the handicap can prevent you from applying the techniques you would use with a normal child. Your handicapped child doesn't need to sleep in your bed any more than other children do; your handicapped child doesn't need to have your company during the night any more than other children do.

Mental handicap

Children who are mentally handicapped are functioning at a more immature level than their actual age, and it is important to keep this in mind when setting expectations for behaviour. Their rate of learning is slower and may be rather idiosyncratic, depending on their problem. You know your child better than anyone else does, and so you need to be alert to how she learns; then you can apply this knowledge to her sleeping pattern.

The most important feature about establishing a regular sleeping pattern is your consistency in management and setting the limits for your child. Very clear routines are essential, so that she learns the difference between day and night, and the pattern of behaviour that you expect at night. Sometimes there is an improvement in sleeping patterns when a child starts playgroup or nursery, as this involves the establishment of a clear daytime routine.

Handicapped children probably have more sleeping problems than normal children. You may feel that there is some neurological difficulty that is causing your child's sleep disturbance. But except in certain very extreme instances, this is not likely, and the majority of mentally handicapped children can be helped to be less disturbed at night.

Richard, a four-year-old autistic boy, had no language and showed marked behaviour problems during the day and at night. He was extremely active, showed no constructive play and required constant adult supervision. His parents lived in a small third-floor council flat, and his mother was six months pregnant when she requested help with his sleeping difficulties. He would not sleep in his own bed, and needed his mother to lie down with him on the parents' bed while he went to sleep. His bedtime was not established, and his mother tended to go to bed with him, because she was anxious not to leave him unsupervised in the bedroom in case he woke up.

He would wake very early in the morning and would generally disrupt the bedroom, pulling off the bedclothes and emptying drawers until his mother got up as well.

Our major concern was to teach Richard to sleep in his own bed in his own room, so that the parents could sleep together undisturbed.

The first step was to make his room totally safe and to put a high-level latch on his door so that he couldn't get out of his room and run around the flat at night.

A bedtime routine was established, with a set bedtime at 7.30 p.m. No graduation of bedtime was thought necessary, as it seemed better to have a definite routine to help him adjust and learn the new pattern. His mother was to settle him to bed in his own room and sit beside him until he fell asleep.

This change in pattern was established within one week

and Richard was falling asleep within a few minutes of having been put to bed. We then planned a gradual withdrawal of mother's presence in the room while he fell asleep, until he could settle himself alone.

During the night, any waking was managed by his mother going into his room and applying the same settling techniques that she was using at bedtime. She agreed that on no account would she take him into her bed. It was a difficult decision, as getting up in the middle of the night was especially tiring while she was pregnant, but she agreed that the long-term benefits would be greater than the short-term discomfort.

Within six weeks Richard was showing a greatly improved sleeping pattern. He went to bed at the set time and would settle to sleep on his own after his bedtime routine. He woke only occasionally at night but could settle to sleep after reassurance.

A spin-off from the improvements was a later rising time with less disruptive behaviour. His parents had put a high latch on the door into the lounge and kitchen area, so he was able to wander around the two bedrooms without needing adult supervision.

This case illustrates the importance of establishing a routine and consistent management as well as trying to deal with disruptive behaviour. After minor practical changes were made, such as high latches on the doors and safety in the bedrooms, Richard's parents did not feel continually anxious when he was out of their sight.

Changes in the amount of parental contact when settling to sleep need to be more gradual than in the straightforward checking approach (see pp. 68–71); but the limits must be firm, so that the child has the opportunity to learn what is expected. Sometimes the speed of change will be slower than for normal children, but this will be determined by your child's level of ability. Be optimistic in your expectations of helping her to settle to sleep, and treat this much as you would teaching her a new skill during the day. Patience, consistency and firm limits are vital.

The visually handicapped child

Getting the blind or partially sighted child to sleep poses difficulties. How can a blind child know when it is dark? How can she learn the signals that it is bedtime? How will she know it is night-time if she wakes up at night? These questions and many more can influence the way in which a normal sighted parent handles a blind child. Feelings of uncertainty about how your child feels and how to give the correct cues for settling to sleep may interrupt a normal pattern of teaching her to sleep on her own. You may develop a pattern of staying with her until she falls asleep more as a reassurance for yourself than for her. The problem then comes when she wakes up in the middle of the night and needs your presence to help her settle again.

A recent small survey has found that, although sleeping problems are very common in severely visually handicapped children, they are not prevalent in residential nurseries; but they are very noticeable at home.[1] The problems were mainly of settling to sleep rather than waking at night.

Simon, a 3½-year-old blind boy, was waking as much as ten times per night and would usually end up sleeping in his parents' bed while his father slept downstairs on the sofa. Simon had developmental and language delay. The family lived in very cramped housing conditions, which forced the parents to have Simon's cot in their bedroom. He had a regular sleeping pattern of going to bed at 6 p.m., sleeping well until about midnight, and then waking. The aim was to help him to sleep in his own bed and to be less disturbed during the night.

The first step was to set a later bedtime, so that Simon's period of sleep happened later. Vallergan forte was prescribed as an aid to this process; it was given at Simon's first waking after 8 p.m. He was encouraged to fall asleep on the sofa downstairs so that the parents could have their bedroom to themselves. This was an interim measure, as the family was due to move to a larger house. The sofa had a sloping seat and back, which cradled Simon safely, and he was supported on one side. It was a familiar place where he would have a daytime nap, and he was physically contained. The parents were reluctant to settle him to sleep in his cot in their room, as they felt that they would be unable to change the habit of his going into their bed.

A graded settling regime was set up, with his mother initially staying with him until he fell asleep; when this was established, she would put on a tape of nursery rhymes for him to listen to while he fell asleep on his own.

Simon adapted well to his new routine, and his sleeping pattern improved greatly. There was a slight setback when the family moved a couple of months later, but after being shown how to find his way round his new house he was settled on the familiar sofa in his new bedroom and gradually transferred to his bed, where he was physically cradled with an eiderdown under him.

One feature of this case which is particularly relevant is the familiarity of the bed or place to sleep; blind children need to feel secure and contained, and the sofa seemed to be ideal with its sloping seat and back. The nursery-rhyme tape uses sound as a mode of comforting in place of a nightlight. Medication was introduced only for a few weeks to allow a shift in the sleeping pattern, because Simon appeared to be getting all of his major sleep before his parents went to bed.

The physically handicapped child

Parents often feel a lot of sorrow and sadness for a physically handicapped child, and they may try to compensate by any means they can. They may feel unwilling to impose any demands on the child, and they often need to talk through their worries and feelings before clear limits for their child's behaviour can be set. It is very easy to want to do things for your handicapped child; leaving it to her can seem cruel and unfair, as physical action is such an effort for her. You may feel guilty and try to take away the problem by working too hard yourselves in an attempt to make life easy for your child.

This happens during the day as well as at night. You know yourself that your child should try to learn to be as independent as possible, but you may feel that rushing up and downstairs with warm drinks during the evening or having a greatly extended bedtime routine is the least you can do. You have a great urge to help and comfort because you know the difficulties your child is facing. But deep inside you know how many problems can arise for your life and your marriage if everything revolves around your child and you as parents have no personal time to yourselves.

Eleanor, a three-year-old spastic girl, showed only a slight delay in her general development, but had very marked sleeping difficulties. She would not go to bed until 11.30 p.m. and then often woke at 2.30 a.m. screaming until she was taken into her parents' bed. She was on Mogadon medication, which made her groggy and tired and had not helped her night-time behaviour.

She could only crawl and had poor sitting balance and limited use of her left arm. Her communication was by pointing and screeching, although her comprehension of language was nearly normal for a three-year-old.

The first step was to stop the medication and set a bedtime routine. Her daytime nap was also reduced from two hours to one. Her mother was encouraged to leave her to settle herself to sleep in the evening; and if Eleanor woke during the night she was to go in and say 'It's still nighttime, go back to sleep.' She would then put on a nursery-rhyme record and leave while Eleanor fell asleep.

Within two weeks there was a great improvement in the sleeping pattern. Eleanor was going to bed by 9.30 p.m., and on 50 per cent of nights she was sleeping through until 8.30 a.m. and had to be woken up. This improvement continued over the next month.

The techniques used in this case are identical with those for normal children described earlier in this book. The setting of a pattern that can be anticipated by the child is important, as well as teaching her to settle to sleep by herself. Eleanor started full-time school at a physically handicapped unit during the time of this intervention, and it is clear that the introduction of school or playgroup often helps handicapped children to accept a newly imposed routine at night. The establishment of clear patterns and routines during the day also appears to affect night-time behaviour.

If your child is multiply handicapped or has one of the various disabilities shown in childhood, then don't give up on sleeping patterns. It is possible to help her to learn more stable and acceptable night-time behaviour. It is difficult enough for you to manage the strain of caring for a handicapped child without the additional stress of never having enough sleep at night. You need your stamina and reserves of strength to get through the day. The worries and concerns will pile up so much more if you are exhausted and irritable through lack of sleep.

Chapter 13
My child wakes early in the morning

Early morning waking can occur with a pattern of disturbed night sleep or as a problem on its own. Many parents just accept that their children wake at 5.30 or 6 a.m. and see it as a natural phase of childhood. This is often true, in that if your child goes to bed at a reasonable time and sleeps well, then he is probably waking at a time when he has had sufficient sleep and is ready for a new day.

Later bedtime

Making bedtime later may make a slight difference to the time when your child wakes, but you need to balance the reduction of your evening against the early start. Many children manage the hour switch from winter to summertime within four or five days, so you can keep this in mind if you want to alter the pattern slightly. This change is possible with children who are generally good sleepers, but does not work so well with poor sleepers. For a poor sleeper, early waking is usually part of the pattern of disturbance, and as your child's night waking is managed differently and reduced you may well find that he also sleeps longer in the morning. This effect seems to be paradoxical but is very common. In 1–2-year-olds, there is also often a increase and greater regularity in daytime naps matching an improvement at night. So in total your child ends up sleeping much more than you ever thought possible, and the routine and generally calmer atmosphere can help him to be less over-excited.

Diverting tactics

It is possible to lengthen the time between your child's waking and his crying to be lifted out of his cot by leaving some interesting toys within his reach or in his cot for him to play with in the morning. Similarly, some parents avoid demands for a drink or a biscuit by leaving them ready beside the child's bed. It is likely that some children are hungry when they wake in the morning.

> Anne, aged 1½, would wake at 6 a.m. but could find the bottle left for her by her mother. She would drink this and then fall asleep again until 8.30 a.m., when her parents got up for work.

It may be easier to keep your child dozing in the early morning if he is still in a cot. The child who can get out of his bed is liable to do so as soon as he wakes up, in order to play with the toys in his room. Some children learn to climb out of their cots at a young age, and it can be dangerous to try to ignore them for a period while you doze. It is easier to get them out and then let them play with some toys in your room while you gradually come round to face the day.

You may feel that you do not want your two-year-old rushing round your bedroom, and that you like to keep one room in the house as a sanctuary where ornaments and personal possessions don't have to be on high shelves out of reach of exploratory fingers. If so, you will probably have to forfeit your lie-in, to get up and be with your child in another room.

The alternative is to have some special toys ready in your bedroom for the morning period while you gently doze. Your child can either get into bed with you for a cuddle or play around on the floor until you are ready to get up.

Encouraging a calm start to the day

One of the worst features of being a parent can be facing a crying child first thing in the morning, particularly if you have had a broken night. Even if you are used to a settled night, a demanding and fractious child first thing can set the day off to a bad start. One possible way round this problem is to get your child up before he starts screaming and crying for you. Many parents are tempted to leave a waking child until he cries, but this teaches him that he has to cry to get attention in the morning. If you can go into the room before this starts and say how pleased you are that he is a happy boy, then everyone feels good. Many preschool children can understand an element of reasoning at this stage, and asking your child not to cry but to call for you may also change the pattern.

Once you feel relatively confident that your child has learned that you will go to him when he is not crying but perhaps playing contentedly in his cot, then it can be possible to leave him a little longer in the morning. This apparently wrong way round of doing things can work well, as your child does not immediately work himself into a frenzy on waking but feels calm and relaxed knowing that at some point you will come in to see him.

Setting a cue for getting up

As we use alarm clocks to wake us up in the morning, it is also possible to use them to indicate to your child when he can come into your room in the morning. This is one way of providing an indication of the suitable time for a 3–4-year-old child. This age-group cannot tell the time, so saying 'Don't come in before seven o'clock' would be meaningless. You might even find your child trotting in every ten minutes from five o'clock on, asking 'Is it seven o'clock yet?' It is also possible to have quite complex discussions about the meaning of 'It's too early' with a lively and inquisitive two-year-old! 'Is it still too early?' can be a question that rebounds through your head as your little girl affectionately does a downstage whisper to the audience right in your ear, while you try to gain just another couple of minutes' sleep.

Alan, a four-year-old, would wake at 5 a.m. most mornings, and his parents decided to try an alarm clock to indicate whether he could go into their room or not. They initially set it for 5.45 a.m., which was the latest time he had woken recently; they were worried that it might wake him up if they set it too early, but that he would not be able to wait for it if it was too late. He was a bright boy and was delighted with his new special clock; and after the first couple of mornings, when he went in to his parents to ask whether it had gone off yet, he settled down quickly into a routine of only going into their room after the alarm. Gradually his parents were able to extend the time by ten-minute stages until the alarm was set for 6.30 a.m., which they felt was a reasonable time for him to start to wake the family.

Tom's father, who was quite a handyman in the home, decided to rig up a system of lights and a time-switch to indicate whether three-year-old Tom could get up and go into his parents' room. The time-switch showed a small red light to indicate that it was too early to get up, and a green light came on at a pre-set time in the morning. For a child who wakes more irregularly, this avoids the risk that an alarm clock might sometimes disturb him when he would have slept on. No parent wants to wake up their child in the morning if it's not necessary! By gradually changing the switch-on time for the green light from 5 a.m. to 7 a.m., Tom's parents were able to gain two more hours of precious sleep.

Rewards and charts

An additional technique that can be used with the ideas mentioned above is to provide a small reward to aid your child's motivation to obey your requests. If he can earn a star or a sticker on a chart for waiting until the alarm goes, then you are likely to gain faster success and change, as it means there is a reward to compete with coming in to you. The new alarm clock alone may not be enough for some children, who will need this extra incentive. There is also the opportunity of immediate feedback for your child's behaviour. It is very important to give the sticker as soon as the alarm has gone. If your child is not interested in a chart, you can provide a small surprise bag which he can dip into for a little present.

It is possible to encourage your child not to disturb you quite so early in the morning, although you are generally unlikely to persuade him to go back to sleep. These techniques are worth a try.

If your child sleeps badly for most of the night as well as waking early, you should work on the night disturbance first; you may find that morning waking resolves itself to an acceptable degree. If not, then it is usually the last part of the disturbed night pattern on which to work.

Chapter 14
Can I help my child to sleep well?

We hope that this book has covered the full range of children's sleep problems and that you will have found at least some advice or an example that is helpful to you.

In our work with severe sleep disturbances, we have been astonished to see the remarkable changes that can be made once parents make up their minds to do something about a problem. Often they have a lot of unspoken anxieties and concerns about how they should manage their child at night. These are very important issues, and it is worthwhile for parents to think them over carefully and to discuss between themselves the issues involved. There is no point in starting to change your approach unless you feel that it is right for you and your child and you know clearly what you are working towards. The advice in this book is not a statement of how we think things should be. The way you choose to respond to your child at night is purely up to you. But if you are unhappy with the present state of affairs it is worth looking carefully at what you might do about it. There are a number of different approaches for each type of problem, so you can choose the style of change that suits you. Try to understand your own feelings, and you will be halfway to understanding the problem. Don't set your sights too high initially, but as you make progress you can increase your expectations of undisturbed evenings and nights.

A possible source of anxiety is a worry that there must be something seriously wrong with your child, otherwise she wouldn't keep waking up or coming down to you. You may fear that there is a physical problem, that she is hyperactive, that she is lacking love, that she is emotionally disturbed or extremely anxious. All these are possibilities, but if your child is growing and developing well and is happy during the day, it is unlikely that she is suffering from anything serious.

If you know that your child has a handicap, it is much harder to decide how to manage her. But, whatever her problem, it will do no harm to be as consistent as possible over night-time management and to encourage a settling routine. This way your child will have as much sleep as possible and you will be rested and can give her more attention during the day.

The main points to take into consideration when preparing to change your management methods are:

1. Have a detailed sleep diary to give you accurate information about the pattern of disturbance and what you are doing.

2. Discuss and agree together what changes you want.

3. Choose an approach to change which suits you and which you feel you could manage.

4. Set yourself small targets if you choose a gradual approach, and wait for complete success at each stage before you progress to the next one.

5. Be consistent. If you decide to react in a certain manner then try to keep to it; but if you can't face the night-time battle tonight, then give in on the first disturbance rather than on the sixth.

6. Back each other up and give support to the one who is taking responsibility for management that night.

7. If you are trying a different approach, then persevere with it for at least four nights before you conclude that it doesn't work. In most cases change will start to be noticeable in this time, if you are being as consistent and firm as you think.

8. Avoid getting into long discussions with your child in the middle of the night about why she is waking. She will only get confused, and she certainly doesn't know the answer.

9. Remember you are the most important person in the world to your child, and if she can't get enough of you during the day, then she will make sure that she does at night.

We aim to give you reassurance about the possibility of improving night-time behaviour in your children without the use of medication. There is a lot of advice around, proffered by friends and relatives as well as by professionals and a wide range of baby and child-care books. This can often be confusing, but the important thing is that you should not be swayed by what other people say they think you should do. You are a parent and have your own special feelings for your child. You can decide perfectly well that what is happening is not suiting you, your child or your marriage. Some families may manage perfectly well with their children falling asleep downstairs and then all sleeping in the parents' bed together, only to wake at five in the morning. If it doesn't suit you, then you can change it; the problem is 'How?' Most of the advice available is based on reasonable premises, but it may be too difficult to face when just dished out as a directive in five minutes. Advice to parents only works if it agrees with an idea already at the back of their mind and fits in well with their feelings.

Amanda, a 2½-year-old, was waking four or five times a night and having a bottle to drink at each waking. The general practitioner had told Amanda's mother to throw away the bottle, which was basically sound advice, but she had been unable to face the prospect of settling her little girl without the bottle available.

In a long discussion this feeling was revealed, and so we examined the possibility of Amanda first learning to fall asleep without her bottle at bedtime before it was later withheld completely during the rest of the night. The mother was very keen to do that, feeling reassured that the bottle was still available for night-time wakings. Within a couple of nights Amanda had accepted falling asleep without it, and would have her drink before getting into bed. We then agreed that since Amanda had stopped having a day-time bottle and her mother now felt confident about the evening, she was ready to stop it at night. Amanda accepted this with no problem at all, and her mother felt quite astonished at how she had become so anxious about the whole issue.

This example demonstrates how important it is to identify your worries about change. You probably already know what you could do to improve matters, but for some reason have not felt able to start. Some parents think their child has a sleeping problem but then find, when they examine their real feelings about change, that they really don't mind her night-time pattern. They are therefore not truly motivated to do anything about it, and it would be inappropriate for them to try.

If you are embarking on a course of change, then remember that your initial aims are to reduce the amount of disturbance to you at night. Your goal is not to get your child to sleep more, though this may happen as a result of her learning not to disturb you. No one knows how long your child should sleep, and we are not stating any expectations in this field. All we can do is to help you have less disturbed nights.

Good luck.

References

Chapter 1

1. **Richman, N.** (1981*a*) 'Sleep problems in young children'. Annotation. *Arch. Dis. Child.* 56, 491–3.
2. **Richman, N., Douglas J., Hunt, H., Levere, R.,** and **Lansdown, R.** (1982) 'Prevalence and treatment of sleep problems in young children'. Paper presented at I.A.C.A.P. Congress, Dublin.

Chapter 2

1. **Kales, A.** (ed.) (1969) *Sleep. Physiology and Pathology. A Symposium.* Philadelphia: J. B. Lippincott.
2. **Anders, T. F.,** and **Guilleminault, C.** (1976) 'The pathophysiology of sleep disorders in pediatrics: I. Sleep in infancy'. *Advances in Pediatrics* 22, 137–50.
3. **Parmelee, A. H., Weiner, N. H.,** and **Schulz, H. R.** (1964) 'Infant sleep patterns from birth to 16 weeks of age'. *J. Pediat.* 65, 576–82.

Chapter 3

1. **Anders, T. F.,** and **Weinstein, P.** (1972) 'Sleep and its disorders in infants and children'. *Pediatrics* 50, 312–24.
2. **Broughton, R.** (1968) 'Sleep disorders: disorders of arousal'. *Science* 159, 1070–77.
3. **Thelen, E.** (1979) 'Rhythmical stereotypes in normal human infants'. *Animal Behaviour* 27, 699–715.
4. **Sallustro, F.,** and **Atwell, C. W.** (1978) 'Body rocking, head banging and head rolling in normal children'. *J. Pediat.* 93, 704–8.
5. **Richman, N.** (1981*b*) 'A community survey of characteristics of one to two year olds with sleep disruptions'. *Am. Acad. Child Psychiat.* 20, 281–91.
6. **Richman, N., Stevenson, J.,** and **Graham, P.** (1975) 'Preva-

lence of behaviour problems in 3 year old children: an epidemiological study in a London borough'. *J. Child Psychol. Psychiat. 16*, 277–87.

Chapter 4

1. **Parmelee, A. H., Weiner, N. H.,** and **Schulz, H. R.** (1964) 'Infant sleep patterns from birth to 16 weeks of age'. *J. Pediat. 65*, 576–82.
2. **Roffwarg, H. P., Dement, W.,** and **Fisher, C.** (1966) 'Ontogenic development of the human sleep dream cycle'. *Science 152*, 604–19.
3. **Moore, T.,** and **Ucko, C.** (1957) 'Night waking in early infancy. Part 1'. *Arch. Dis. Child. 33*, 333–42.
4. **Bernal, J. F.** (1972) 'Crying during the first 10 days of life and maternal responses'. *Dev. Med. Child Neurol. 14*, 362–72.
5. **Kitzinger, M.,** and **Hunt, H.** (1982) 'The effect of residential setting on sleep and behaviour patterns of young visually handicapped children'. Paper presented at I.A.C.A.P. Congress, Dublin.
6. **Tucker, I. G.,** and **McArthur, K.** (1977) 'The sleep patterns of preschool hearing impaired children'. *J. Br. Assoc. Teachers Deaf 1*, 2–7.
7. **Hide, D. W.,** and **Guyer, B. M.** (1982) 'Prevalence of infant colic'. *Arch. Dis. Child. 57*, 559–60.
8. **Minford, A. M. B., MacDonald, A.,** and **Littlewood, J. M.** (1982) 'Food intolerance and food allergy in children: a review of 68 cases'. *Arch. Dis. Child. 57*, 742–47.
9. **Evans, R. W.,** *et al.* (1981) 'Maternal diet and infantile colic in breast fed infants'. *Lancet 1*, 1340–42.
10. **Weiss, B.** (1982) 'Food additives and environmental chemicals as sources of childhood behavior disorders'. *J. Amer. Acad. Child Psychiat. 21*, 144–52.
11. **Taylor, E.** (1979) 'Food additives, allergy and hyperkinesis'. Annotation. *J. Child Psychol. Psychiat. 20*, 357–64.
12. **Richman, N.** (1981*b*) 'A community survey of characteristics of one to two year olds with sleep disruptions'. *Am. Acad. Child Psychiat. 20*, 281–91.

13. **Blurton-Jones, N.,** *et al.* (1978) 'The association between perinatal factors and later night waking'. *Dev. Med. Child Neurol.* 20, 427–34.

14. **Bernal, J.** (1973) 'Night waking in infants during the first 14 months'. *Dev. Med. Child Neurol.* 15, 760–69.

15. **Carey, W.** (1974) 'Night waking and temperament in infancy'. *J. Pediat.* 84, 756–8.

16. **Sander, L.,** *et al.* (1970) 'Early mother-infant interactions and 24 hour patterns of activity and sleep'. *J. Amer. Acad. Child Psychiat.* 9, 103–23.

17. **Brackbill, Y.** (1973) 'Continuous stimulation reduces arousal level: stability of the effects over time'. *Child Dev.* 44, 43–6.

18. **Chisholm, J. S.,** and **Richards, M. P. M.** (1978) 'Swaddling, cradleboards and the development of children'. *Early Human Develop.* 2, 255–75.

19. **Lipton, E., Steinschneider, A.,** and **Richmond, J.** (1965) 'Swaddling: a child care practice'. *Pediatrics* 35, 519–67.

20. **Ozturk, M.,** and **Ozturk, O. M.** (1977) 'Thumb-sucking and falling asleep'. *Brit. J. Med. Psychol.* 50, 95–103.

21. **Yarrow, L. J.** (1954) 'The relationship between nutritive experiences in infancy and non-nutritive sucking in childhood.' *J. Genet. Psychol.* 84, 149–62.

22. **Passman, R. H.,** and **Halonen, J. S.** (1979) 'A developmental survey of young children's attachments to inanimate objects'. *J. Genet. Psychol.* 134, 165–78.

23. **Boniface, D.,** and **Graham, P.** (1979) 'The three year old child and his attachment to a special soft object'. *J. Child Psychol. Psychiat.* 20, 217–24.

Chapter 5

1. **Caudill, W.,** and **Plath, D. W.** (1966) 'Who sleeps by whom? Parent-child involvement in urban Japanese families'. *Psychiatry* 29, 344–66.

2. **Richman, N.** (1981b) 'A community survey of characteristics of one to two year olds with sleep disruptions'. *Am. Acad. Child Psychiat.* 20, 281–91.

3. **Thomas, A.**, *et al.* (1963) *Behavioral Individuality in Early Childhood.* New York: N.Y. University Press.

Chapter 6
1. **Ounstead, M. K.**, and **Hendrick, A. M.** (1977) 'The first born child: patterns of development'. *Dev. Med. Child Neurol. 19,* 446–53.

Chapter 12
1. **Kitzinger, M.**, and **Hunt, H.** (1982) 'The effect of residential setting on sleep and behaviour patterns of young visually handicapped children'. Paper presented at I.A.C.A.P. Congress, Dublin.

Index

READ MORE IN PENGUIN

In every corner of the world, on every subject under the sun, Penguin represents quality and variety – the very best in publishing today.

For complete information about books available from Penguin – including Puffins, Penguin Classics and Arkana – and how to order them, write to us at the appropriate address below. Please note that for copyright reasons the selection of books varies from country to country.

In the United Kingdom: Please write to *Dept. JC, Penguin Books Ltd, FREEPOST, West Drayton, Middlesex UB7 0BR*

If you have any difficulty in obtaining a title, please send your order with the correct money, plus ten per cent for postage and packaging, to *PO Box No. 11, West Drayton, Middlesex UB7 0BR*

In the United States: Please write to *Penguin USA Inc., 375 Hudson Street, New York, NY 10014*

In Canada: Please write to *Penguin Books Canada Ltd, 10 Alcorn Avenue, Suite 300, Toronto, Ontario M4V 3B2*

In Australia: Please write to *Penguin Books Australia Ltd, 487 Maroondah Highway, Ringwood, Victoria 3134*

In New Zealand: Please write to *Penguin Books (NZ) Ltd,182–190 Wairau Road, Private Bag, Takapuna, Auckland 9*

In India: Please write to *Penguin Books India Pvt Ltd, 706 Eros Apartments, 56 Nehru Place, New Delhi 110 019*

In the Netherlands: Please write to *Penguin Books Netherlands B.V., Keizersgracht 231 NL–1016 DV Amsterdam*

In Germany: Please write to *Penguin Books Deutschland GmbH, Friedrichstrasse 10–12, W–6000 Frankfurt/Main 1*

In Spain: Please write to *Penguin Books S. A., C. San Bernardo 117–6° E–28015 Madrid*

In Italy: Please write to *Penguin Italia s.r.l., Via Felice Casati 20, I–20124 Milano*

In France: Please write to *Penguin France S. A., 17 rue Lejeune, F–31000 Toulouse*

In Japan: Please write to *Penguin Books Japan, Ishikiribashi Building, 2–5–4, Suido, Tokyo 112*

In Greece: Please write to *Penguin Hellas Ltd, Dimocritou 3, GR–106 71 Athens*

In South Africa: Please write to *Longman Penguin Southern Africa (Pty) Ltd, Private Bag X08, Bertsham 2013*